BODIES THAT BIRTH

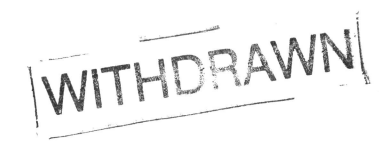

Bodies that Birth puts birthing bodies at the center of questions about contemporary birth politics, power and agency. Arguing that the fleshy and embodied aspects of birth have been largely silenced in social science scholarship, Rachelle Chadwick uses an array of birth stories, from diverse race–class demographics, to explore the narrative entanglements between flesh, power and sociomateriality in relation to birth.

Adopting a unique theoretical framework incorporating new materialism, feminist theory and a Foucauldian 'analytics of power,' the book aims to trace and trouble taken-for-granted assumptions about birthing bodies. Through a diffractive and dialogical approach, the analysis highlights the interplay between corporeality, power and ideologies in the making of birth narratives across a range of intersectional differences. The book shows that there is no singular birthing body apart from sociomaterial relations of power. Instead, birthing bodies are uncertain zones or unpredictable assortments of physiology, flesh, sociomateriality, discourse and affective flows. At the same time, birthing bodies are located within intra-acting fields of power relations, including biomedicine, racialized patriarchy, socioeconomics and geopolitics.

Bodies that Birth brings the voices of women from different sociomaterial positions into conversation. Ultimately, the book explores how attending to birthing bodies can vitalize global birth politics by listening to what matters to women in relation to birth. This is fascinating reading for researchers, academics and students from across the social sciences.

Rachelle Chadwick is NRF Research Career Fellow in the Gender Studies Section of the School of African and Gender Studies, Anthropology and Linguistics at the Univers

WOMEN AND PSYCHOLOGY

Series Editor: Jane Ussher
Professor of Women's Health Psychology, University of Western Sydney

This series brings together current theory and research on women and psychology. Drawing on scholarship from a number of different areas of psychology, it bridges the gap between abstract research and the reality of women's lives by integrating theory and practice, research and policy.

Each book addresses a 'cutting edge' issue of research, covering topics such as postnatal depression and eating disorders, and addressing a wide range of theories and methodologies.

The series provides accessible and concise accounts of key issues in the study of women and psychology, and clearly demonstrates the centrality of psychology debates within women's studies or feminism.

Other titles in this series:

'Adolescence', Pregnancy and Abortion
Catriona I. Macleod

The Madness of Women
Jane M. Ussher

Fat Lives
Irmgard Tischner

Knowing Victims
Rebecca Stringer

The Psychological Development of Girls and Women
Second edition
Sheila Greene

Adopted Women and Biological Fathers
Elizabeth Hughes

BODIES THAT BIRTH

Vitalizing Birth Politics

Rachelle Chadwick

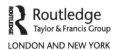
Routledge
Taylor & Francis Group

LONDON AND NEW YORK

First published 2018
by Routledge
2 Park Square, Milton Park, Abingdon, Oxon OX14 4RN

and by Routledge
711 Third Avenue, New York, NY 10017

Routledge is an imprint of the Taylor & Francis Group, an informa business

© 2018 Rachelle Chadwick

British Library Cataloguing-in-Publication Data
A catalogue record for this book is available from the British Library

Library of Congress Cataloging-in-Publication Data
A catalog record for this book has been requested

ISBN: 978-1-138-12333-5 (hbk)
ISBN: 978-1-138-12334-2 (pbk)
ISBN: 978-1-315-64891-0 (ebk)

Typeset in Bembo
by Swales & Willis Ltd. Exeter, Devon, UK

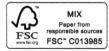

MIX
Paper from
responsible sources
FSC
www.fsc.org   FSC™ C013985

Printed in the United Kingdom
by Henry Ling Limited

For Barry Chadwick
January 2, 1939–July 21, 2015
My deepest inspiration in life and work.

CONTENTS

Acknowledgments   viii
List of abbreviations   x

1   Opening   1

2   Birthing bodies: the politics of framing   24

3   Clockwork bodies   50

4   Risky bodies   73

5   Violated bodies   102

6   Resistant bodies   131

7   What matters? Vitalizing birth politics   170

8   Closing   200

References   204
Appendix 1: Research note   219
Appendix 2: Transcription notation   222
Index   223

ACKNOWLEDGMENTS

This book is the culmination of a long intellectual and personal journey, spanning many years, academic departments, relationships and places. The journey was not linear or neatly progressive but punctuated with loss, self-doubt and disappointment. These acknowledgments are written primarily for those, both human and animal, that supported, loved and affirmed me through many difficult and challenging times.

First, I wish to thank and acknowledge the 64 women that shared their lives and motherhood journeys with me—without them this book could not exist. Thank you for your generosity of spirit and for gifting me with your precious stories. Thank you also to those that facilitated the recruitment process. In particular I wish to thank the staff and community counsellors at The Parent Centre and various private midwives working in the greater Cape Town area for their assistance and support.

I also want to thank the many teachers and mentors that crisscrossed through my life and inspired me over the years in different ways (mostly without knowing it) including: Tammy Shefer, Andy Dawes, Sally Swartz, Diane Cooper, Jane Bennett and Trinh Minh-ha. Thank you for intellectual inspiration, collegial support and for your discernable and inspiring commitment—to work, ideas and ethics. It has not gone unnoticed.

The empirical work on which this book is based was conducted while I was a PhD student in the Psychology Department and a Postdoctoral Fellow in the Women's Health Research Unit at the University of Cape Town (UCT). The book was, however, written while based in the Gender Studies Section of the School of African and Gender Studies, Anthropology and Linguistics at UCT. Thank you to my colleagues in the Gender Studies Section for providing a warm and supportive 'home' and allowing me the space I needed to write and to think.

Thank you to the Series Editor, Jane Ussher, for seeing merit in my project early on and for encouraging me to write this book. Appreciation and thanks are also extended to the anonymous reviewers who commented on early versions of this book. Thank you also to the editing staff at Routledge for their work on the book, kind assistance and patience!

I have been the fortunate recipient of generous funding and financial assistance from a number of sources, including the A.W. Mellon Foundation, the National Research Foundation (NRF) and the University of Cape Town. Without this support, this book would not have been written. In particular, I wish to acknowledge and thank the NRF for the generous Research Career Advancement Fellowship that was awarded to me in 2014. Thank you for showing faith in my research at a difficult time and supporting my intellectual work and growth as an academic.

My heartfelt thanks to my mother for her endless support and love—and for the hours she spent knitting baby jackets for several of the women who participated in the project. It is your incredible strength and commitment as a mother that has inspired my ongoing interest in women's reproductive, mothering and care work. The book is dedicated to my father who passed away on 21 July 2015. He was and still is a powerful presence in my life, providing me with a strong moral and ethical compass and a remarkable example of a life lived with integrity, courage, hope and honesty. I looked to my father for inspiration when writing this book and I found it. It was only through his example that I found the strength and willpower to get up morning after morning at 5 a.m. to write.

I would like to thank and acknowledge Don—basically, *for everything*. Thank you for being the most amazing and inspiring teacher—in your passion for ideas I found a kindred spirit. You have inspired me in every possible way and this book is a culmination not only of my work and thinking but of our joint journey. Thank you for believing in my work and supporting me through injury, illness, death and disappointment. I thank you—with all of me. Thank you also to our most beloved animal companions—Lulu, Mimi, Stornie, Robbie, Picksy-Malinka and others (some departed from this world) who have befriended me and warmed my life over the years. Your loyalty, generosity, unconditional love and purity of spirit give me hope and always manage to renew me when life becomes challenging or painful.

Lastly, I wish to thank you, the reader, for engaging with my words and this book. I hope that the stories and voices within it move you, make you think and speak to you in productive ways. I apologize for any gaffes I have made or shortcomings in the book (which are undoubtedly there and entirely my own). My sincere hope is, however, that this book becomes a kind of friend to you (as so many have become for me) and finds a cozy spot on your shelf.

ABBREVIATIONS

CDC	Centers for Disease Prevention and Contol
EFM	electronic foetal monitor
FREDA	fairness, respect, equality, dignity and autonomy
GDP	gross domestic product
MMR	maternal mortality rate
MOU	Maternal Obstetric Unit
NGO	non-governmental organization
PTSD	post-traumatic stress disorder
WHO	World Health Organization

1

OPENING

This book is about the fleshy politics of birthing bodies. To begin, it might be pertinent to ask: why this book? Do we need a book about bodies, birth and politics? It is well known that feminists and social scientists have studied birth extensively over the last 40 years. As a result, there is abundant research on the topic. And while bodies were theoretically sexy in the 1990s (see Frank, 1990), surely they are out of fashion by now? My argument is that while a substantial corpus of research has investigated birth and there has been widespread engagement with 'the body' and corporeality in the social sciences, there has been little research that has engaged with *birthing bodies*. Social science researchers have been largely silent about the possible political, ethical and theoretical implications and meanings of birthing embodiment (Walsh, 2010) and have tended to ignore the fleshy materiality of birth as a topic of empirical investigation. This is interesting given that substantial attention has been paid to other aspects of procreative embodiment (i.e. pregnancy, breastfeeding and maternity). Despite the undeniably 'fleshy' and corporeal aspects of giving birth, researchers have been reluctant to engage with birth *as a bodily event.*

My argument in this book is that *this silence matters* and tells us something about the ontological politics of birth. I will argue that it points to dualist understandings of the body that births in feminist, biomedical, midwifery and social science writing and debate. Furthermore, while birthing bodies are rarely directly addressed, problematized or theorized, assumptions about the nature of these bodies pervade medical, activist and social science discourse. Birthing bodies are thus paradoxically both absent and omnipresent. In this book, I explore ontological framings of the body that births in feminist and social science research, as well as in broader birth debates among midwives, activists, birth workers, practitioners and feminists. I will argue that many of these framings are problematic, limited and a poor basis for trying to imagine positive, affirming and alternative ways of doing birth.

In particular, I argue that the failure to engage critically with birthing bodies has limited feminist debate, research and birth activism/s. Furthermore, narrow, dualist and homogenous assumptions about birthing bodies has limited our (feminist) ability to understand, conceptualize and ultimately improve, women's birth experiences.

We are currently witnessing a period of stagnation in relation to the feminist politics of birth, particularly in Northern settings, which has been argued to be currently characterized by conceptual impasses (see Walsh, 2010) and limited by narrow neoliberal valorizations of 'choice' (Beckett, 2005). The lack of engagement with the embodied, fleshy and intersectional ontologies and politics of birth has resulted in lack of clarity about what matters in relation to birth and misrecognition of the geopolitical and sociomaterial aspects of birth politics. Continued essentialist understandings of birthing bodies and pervasive mind–body dualism have limited our ability to conceptualize and fully hear what women are saying when they tell stories about their births. Furthermore, narrow binary conceptualizations of bio-medical versus natural models of birth, usually written from privileged geopolitical positions, has stymied our ability to think of birth in alternative, heterogeneous and intersectional ways. This book puts birthing bodies at the center of questions about birth politics, intersectionality, agency, resistance and power relations and ultimately argues that engagement with the complexity of birthing embodiment has the potential to vitalize the feminist politics of birth and open new directions for birth activism and scholarship.

Why bodies, birth and politics?

This book is about birth, bodies and politics. The *politics* I am interested in is not the ordinary kind to be found in the daily newspaper or on the evening news. Instead, it is a politics interested in questions of representation and framing, as well as everyday, embodied enactments of inequality. This is *ontological politics* (Mol, 2002). According to Mol (2002, p. viii), ontological politics involves tracing, "the way in which problems are framed, bodies are shaped, and lives are pushed and pulled." This involves exploring the ways material-discursive framings are enacted, negotiated, lived and resisted by embodied persons in everyday practices and events. It is the ontological politics of birth that I focus on in this book. Women's birth narratives are used as openings from which to explore the corporeal politics of birth as played out in the South African setting and beyond.

Alongside ontological politics, I also focus on *birthing bodies*. It is my argument that birthing bodies are good to think with. Focusing on birthing bodies throws the politics of birth into sharp relief, revealing lines of flight between transnational birth debates, global/local inequalities, technocratic norms, ideological story lines and women's embodied birthing experiences. The birthing bodies that will mate-rialize over the pages of this book will be multiple and emergent, morphing into different shapes according to the play of ontological birth politics and sociomaterial positionings. Bodies are understood as sociomaterialities: assorted jumbles of fleshy physiology, discourse, history, techno-science, tools, machines, intersubjective relations and space-time politics. These are bodies shaped by multiple forces and yet they are also capacities able to act, affect, respond, resist and interact. Birthing bodies are not stable givens but uncertain zones that materialize and act in relation to an entanglement of crosscutting forces. There is no singular birthing body. Birth is never a matter just of physiology, biology or even culture. Birth is always embedded, emergent and *in relation to* sociocultural norms, local material structures, physiologies, intersectional and transnational relations of power. Birth is situated at the crossroads of body, sociomateriality, physiology, discourse, language and geopolitics. The birthing body is not one. Multiple birthing bodies become—materialize—through sociomaterial enactments and shifting ontological, epistemological and political framings.

To capture birthing bodies as complex, multiple and emergent entanglements, I draw on a range of theoretical and methodological resources and concepts in this book, including: Michel Foucault's 'analytics of power'; new materialist concepts of assemblage, diffraction and intra-action; Julia Kristeva's theorization of the relationship between language and bodies; and a dialogical approach to narratives (Frank, 2010). These theories, approaches and concepts are used diffractively (Barad, 2007) to trace birthing bodies as multiplicities that are not stable but materialize as/within fields of *relatings* between diffracting voices, practices and sociomaterialities. Birthing bodies have no singular or essential nature; they are fluid and permeable energies and capacities that become in relation to sociomaterial ensembles. Birthing bodies are thus not just represented by discourses—they are literally 'made up' (they become) via diffractive play between physiologies, space-time politics, discourses and sociomaterial inequalities.

Why now?

This book is written at a time when the global and local politics of birth are contested. According to Reiger and Dempsey (2006, p. 364) there is a "sense of crisis" about birth in the twenty-first century. Rising rates of biomedical intervention and caesarean section (across South/North divides), the hegemony of risk discourse, high rates of unnecessary maternal deaths in many Southern contexts, increasing reports of (predominantly Northern) women being distressed and 'traumatized' after birth and the growing clamor of birth activists naming obstetric violence as a global health problem, all speak to a current series of explosive tensions circulating in and around birth. In Northern contexts, pervasive biomedical risk discourse coexists with neoliberal tendencies towards the individualization of responsibility and a consumer approach to birth. Women are thus ostensibly free to make individual 'choices' about birth while the overdetermination and ontological politics of these choices is often overlooked. As a result, some women in Northern contexts are left wondering about the disjuncture between their birth plan and their lived experience. For example, reflecting on her own highly medicalized birth experience, feminist psychologist Michele Crossley (2007, p. 559) laments, "I still do not know if I should be challenging medicalization or not."

Along with the construction of birth as a biomedically risky event, there is also (paradoxically) intensive idealization of so-called physiological or 'normal' birth (see Rossiter, 2017; Vissing, 2017), particularly among middle-class, privileged women in Northern contexts. As a result, many middle-class women are left feeling like 'failures' (as women, as mothers) after birth via caesarean section. In the North, psychological distress, unhappiness and 'trauma' are widely reported by women after birth. Studies have found that more than one third of women in these contexts report their births to have been traumatic (see Creedy, Shochet & Horsfall, 2000; Soet, Brack & Dilorio, 2003; Baker, Choi & Henshaw, 2005; Olde et al., 2005). For privileged women in the Global North, birth is as safe as it has ever been but many women are unhappy with their birth experiences. For marginalized (i.e. immigrant, black, disabled, queer, trans) women in Northern settings, birth is clouded by social injustices stemming from a range of intersecting inequalities. For example, racial inequalities in the USA materialize viscerally as embodied inequalities during pregnancy and birth with evidence of substantial disparities in maternal mortality rates for black and white women. For example, according to data from the Centers for Disease Prevention and Control (CDC), black women are more than three times more likely to die during birth than white women in the USA (Pregnancy Mortality Surveillance System, 2016). Such embodied inequalities are also visible on a global scale, with maternal mortality rates differing radically according to geopolitical zones (i.e. North/South). For example, while in sub-Saharan Africa there is a 1 in 36 lifetime risk of dying during birth, in high-income contexts the risk is 1 in 4,900 (The Lancet Series, 2016). While many women are unhappy with their births in high-income contexts, in the Global South, unacceptable numbers of women are still dying during pregnancy and birth. Furthermore, there is increasing dissatisfaction with the 'care' that women receive during birth and labor in a range of different settings and across North/South divides. While more than one third of women are left feeling 'traumatized' after birth in high-income contexts, there is evidence of widespread abuse, mistreatment and the violation of women's human rights (to respect, informed consent and confidentiality) in many Southern contexts. In a global sense, all is not well with birth. Many women are unhappy with their experiences and pregnancy/birth remains a central locus for the reiteration of social inequalities, both locally and on a transnational scale.

Why here?

South Africa is a middle-income country of the geopolitical 'South,' with a long history of colonial oppression, racial injustice/s and apartheid. Despite the transition to democracy in 1994, South Africa continues to be a highly divided society plagued by violence, poverty and racial tensions. It is also one of the most consistently unequal societies in the world, with a Gini coefficient of approximately 0.69 (StatsSA, 2014). Birth politics are inextricably shaped by these sociomaterial inequalities and historical legacies. The health system, in particular, continues to be plagued by the aftermath of apartheid and racial inequalities that materialize as sharp differences in health infrastructure and resources between the state-funded public sector and the private health care sector (only accessible to those with private medical aids). Approximately 8 percent of gross domestic product (GDP) is spent on health care in South Africa (Econex, 2013). Despite a relatively even split in the expenditure of these resources between the public and private health care sectors, the public sector provides health care to approximately 83 percent of the population while the private sector supports only about 17 percent of South Africans (South African Demographic and Health Survey, 2007). As a result, approximately 50 percent of health expenditure is directed towards a privileged, predominantly white minority. It is estimated that approximately 84 percent of white South African women have access to private sector health care compared to 32 percent of black African women (StatsSA, 2013). While the private health care system has advanced infrastructure, state of the art technology and a high proportion of highly skilled medical specialists, the public sector languishes with poor infrastructure, lack of resources, staff and available medical technology.

This results in vastly different pregnancy and birth experiences for South African women in relation to class/race positions given that the public/private split is still highly racialized (see StatsSA, 2013). As a result, most of the 83 percent of patients using public sector services in South Africa are black and poor (South African Demographic and Health Survey, 2007). While both public and private maternal health care systems are medicalized, with 96 percent of South African women giving birth in a health care facility (South African Demographic and Health Survey, 2017), birth materializes differently according to public/private institutional dynamics. Local maternal mortality rates (MMRs) reflect these differences and inequalities, with the MMR in the private sector estimated as 40 deaths per 100,000 live births (Bateman, 2014), while in the public sector the estimate is approximately 333 deaths per 100,000 live births (Bradshaw, Dorrington & Laubscher, 2012). Women in the public sector are thus approximately eight times more likely to die because of pregnancy-/birth-related complications than privileged women accessing private health care. Inequalities are powerfully inscribed on birthing bodies in the South African context, sometimes with life/death consequences. Rates of caesarean section and medical intervention also follow different trajectories in South Africa according to private/public sector dynamics. Caesarean sections are extremely high in the private sector, with estimates ranging between 40 and 82 percent (Rothberg & Macleod, 2005; Tshibangu et al., 2002; Naidoo & Moodley, 2009). In the public sector, the rate of caesarean sections is estimated as between 15 and 20 percent. However, certain tertiary level academic hospitals reportedly have higher caesarean section rates. For example, Chris Hani Baragwanath, one of the largest tertiary hospitals in South Africa, is estimated as having a caesarean section rate of 39 percent (Ayob, 2014).

Despite health care reforms implemented over the last 20 years, such as the provision of free antenatal care and obstetric services to all women, South Africa continues to have unacceptably high MMR's, which have not decreased sufficiently since 1990 (Bradshaw & Dorrington, 2012). In fact, MMR's reportedly increased in the period between 1990 and 2010 from approximately 150 deaths per 100,000 births in 1990 to around 625 deaths per 100,000 births in 2010 (Blaauw & Penn-Kekana, 2010). However, from 2010 onwards, MMR's have reportedly been in decline (Moodley et al., 2014). While HIV/AIDS is still a significant indirect cause of maternal mortality in the South African context, approximately 59 percent of deaths are due to direct causes (i.e. hypertension, maternal hemorrhage, maternal sepsis, obstructed labor and abortion) that are preventable with good quality health care. Reports of mistreatment, violence and the violation of basic human rights are widespread in the public maternal health sector (see Jewkes, Abrahams & Mvo, 1998; Rattner et al., 2007; Van den Broek & Graham, 2009; Kruger & Schoombie, 2010; Mathai, 2011; Chadwick, Cooper & Harries, 2014; Chadwick, 2016). There have, as yet, not been studies exploring possible mistreatment/s within the private sector. The excessively high caesarean section rates, however, point towards over-medicalization as a substantial problem in private health care settings.

Giving birth in South Africa is thus not a neutral, uncomplicated affair, nor is it only an individual matter or 'experience.' Birth is intertwined with broader body politics and social inequalities. In South Africa, birth politics are bifurcated and straddle both abnormally high levels of medicalization and caesarean section (for privileged women) and neglect, mistreatment, poor quality of care and high maternal mortality rates for low-income women. As a result, the South African context is reflective of many of the current global controversies surrounding birth, including: rising medicalization, bioeconomic neoliberalism and the politics of 'choice,' birth violence and mistreatment and complex entanglements between positions of privilege and marginalization and materializations of birth. South Africa thus offers a rich context in which to explore the ontological and corporeal politics of birth as played out in relation to geopolitics, race–class dynamics and gender politics. South Africa is a strange mix of high-tech and highly specialist obstetrics, neoliberal politics and bioeconomics, privilege and wealth *and* extreme poverty, lack of resources, Southern geopolitics and a deficient public maternal health care sector. As a result, it is a microcosm mirroring broader North–South bifurcations and offers an opportunity to explore the politics of birth from a Southern feminist perspective. This is important given that most feminist analyses of birth have been written from Northern geopolitical zones and have centered the experiences of privileged, Euro-American women.

Using a racially and socioeconomically diverse group of 64 South African women's birth narratives as 'data,' this book focuses on birthing bodies, ontological politics and the entangled modes of power and resistance produced in birth storytelling (see Appendix 1 for further details). Most feminist social science research on birth has been conducted with middle-class, privileged groups of women in 'Northern' geopolitical contexts. The feminist politics of birth has thus been dominated by the concerns and experiences of privileged women. As a result, many concepts and factors that have been extensively explored in relation to birth, including 'control,' 'choice,' trauma, the critique of biomedicalization and the idealization and endorsement of 'natural childbirth,' are predicated on the concerns of women in the Global North. Unfortunately, this is often not acknowledged and the perspectives of privileged women are often treated as decontextualized universals. Literature on women's birth experiences in Southern contexts has followed a different set of trajectories. Scholarship and birth activism in Latin American contexts has been dominated over the last two decades by the critique of biomedicalization and the development of the concept of 'obstetric violence' (Pérez D' Gregorio, 2010). In African contexts, literature on birth has been dominated by public health research and predominantly been concerned with issues of maternal mortality and morbidity and abusive treatment. African women's birth narratives have not been widely explored. In many senses, there is thus a bifurcation in birth scholarship in which research on privileged, middle-class women in Northern settings and 'marginalized' women in the Global South, and Africa in particular, continue to develop and exist as separate literatures. Situated in the South African context that straddles boundaries between privilege and marginalization, 'First World' and 'Third World' realities, this book draws on material that attempts to trouble taken-for-granted bifurcations and binaries. The analysis moves between and across the birth stories of women situated in diverse race, class and sociomaterial positions. The stories of privileged (often white) South African women birthing in high-tech settings, and low-income, sociomaterially marginalized black women birthing in state-funded and under-resourced settings, are put into conversation.

A key aim of this book is to explore the multivocality of birth narratives across these sociomaterial divides and contestations. The goal is not just to explore individual narratives but also to position them in relation to ontological and intersectional body politics. My aim is to represent women (as they tell birth) as ambiguous, intersectional, embodied subjects caught in a sticky web of power relations, sliding between acts of resistance, compliance, passivity and collusion. This book is thus about the birthing bodies reproduced in women's birth narratives, but it is also about the messy, slippery relations between power, politics, agency, positionality, desire and resistance. Central to the exploration of these sliding relations is the matter of bodies. Recognized by some theorists as, "the crucial term" (Grosz, 1994, p. 19) in debates about power, agency and subjectivity, the book argues that thinking through and with birthing bodies is critical in efforts both to understand the full complexity of women's birth narratives and vitalize the feminist politics of birth. Given the focus on conceptualizing birthing bodies, theoretical frames are of critical importance to my project. In the following section, I discuss the theoretical influences that inform and shape my analytic approach in this book.

Theoretical entanglements

My work is shaped by a number of theoretical frames. A social constructionist approach to subjectivities, 'realities' and power relations (Haslanger, 2012; Burr, 2015) serves as one key point of departure. In constructionism, social life and norms are regarded as fundamentally shaped and constructed by language games, discursive frames and interpretative histories. Stories, accounts and talk are not seen as reflections of authentic experience or unchanging, pure 'reality' but are themselves enabled by broader discourses, circulating sociocultural representations and cultural narratives. However, my work is also situated in a relation of tension with social constructionist assumptions about bodies and materiality. Social constructionist frameworks, while offering important insights about the discursive social production of 'experience,' everyday truths and sociocultural forms of life, sometimes fall short when it comes to thinking through the material, fleshy and bodily aspects of subjectivity and sociality (Hekman, 2010; Chadwick, 2017a). Social constructionist approaches can be guilty of disembodying selves and reproducing them as empty discursive fictions, fragmented and without substance. Matter and bodies often materialize only as static bedrocks or blank templates for social and discursive inscription. New materialist approaches (see DeLanda, 2006; Barad, 2007; Alaimo & Hekman, 2008; Alaimo, 2010; Coole & Frost, 2010; Pitts-Taylor, 2016) have developed as a result of increasing frustration with the limited framework/s social constructionism offers vis-à-vis the theorization of materiality, matter, the non-human and fleshy bodies. While I will be drawing on new materialism in this book, my approach is also strongly influenced by a Foucauldian reading of bodies and their relationship to power.

Foucauldian bodies and power relations

Within constructionist frameworks, bodies are conceptualized as social texts inscribed by sociocultural practices, power relations and normative discourses. In this approach, there is no natural or essential body that is knowable or separate from culture. Bodies are understood as passive templates that materialize in relation to linguistic and discursive frames (McLaren, 2002). As a result, theorists argue that there is no pre-discursive body intelligible outside of social discourse (Butler, 1993; Gatens, 1996). While some deny that he was ever a poststructuralist (see Hekman, 2010), the work of Michel Foucault (1979) has been particularly influential in thinking through the relations between bodies, power and discourse.

In Foucauldian theory, bodies emerge as the key objects and targets of modern forms of power, which work via surveillance, institutionalization, categorization, normalizing tactics and regimes of discipline to 'inscribe' and produce 'docile bodies' (Foucault, 1979). Bodies are seen as the products of power relations, which involves both discursive inscription (i.e. interpellative norms) and material practices (Hekman, 2010). According to Foucault, modern power is no longer synonymous with oppression, domination or repression (although it does sometimes include such relations). Power is instead reconceived as productive and constitutive of selves, bodies and desires, as microanalytic rather than totalizing, and spread capillary-like throughout the social field. Power is also not necessarily only a force or form of coercion that is imposed on the subject from the outside. Disciplinary power operates via normalization, the creation of hierarchies and material mechanisms of surveillance and visibility that become naturalized. When most productive, disciplinary power becomes internalized as forms of self-discipline and self-policing;

the subject essentially becomes "the principle of his own subjection" (Foucault, 1979, p. 203). Disciplinary power thus does not only work to reduce, constrain, coerce or restrict but also enables, generates, produces capabilities, creates desires, shapes actions and constructs identities. As such there can be no pure 'experience,' personal choice, body, story or event that is *separate* from relations of power. While Foucault is often characterized as theorizing the body as constructed by discourses, his work on power is far more sophisticated and engages with questions of how to think through the relations between discourse and materiality or 'words and things' (Hekman, 2010). Foucault offers a dynamic and fluid theory of the materialization of bodies as occurring via practices, techniques and strategies of power. Power is not a 'thing' but a relation; it is also not separate from resistance. Power acts on the body but the body also articulates power; this is a relational dynamic that is thoroughly corporeal.

Foucault's conceptualization of power will be crucial to the analysis in this book. The birthing bodies represented in women's birth narratives will not be regarded as authentic reflections of unmediated bodily experiences. Instead, the ways in which women speak about birth and tell stories are regarded as framed by broader socio-cultural interpretive repertoires and cultural narratives. Power relations are seen as a productive and constructive force that leaks, mingles with and shapes birth narratives and women's embodied experiences of birth. Traditional conceptions of power in birth scholarship often assume power to be solely 'top-down' and oppressive. In particular, biomedical power has often been cast as inherently disem-powering and exploitative in relation to birth (i.e. Oakley, 1980; Rothman, 1982). While more recent feminist work has moved away from the 'biomedicalization equals oppression' thesis and acknowledged that many privileged Euro-American women actively desire and are even empowered by biomedical modes of birth (see Davis-Floyd, 2003; Fox & Worts, 1999), for the most part feminist scholarship is still limited by models of power that posit clear distinctions between power, structure, ideology and the individual subject. As a result, the finding that many middle-class, privileged women in the Global North desire biomedicalized modes of birth is often treated as transparent evidence of women's 'agency' or personal 'choice.'

The entangled relations between desire, choice and power have not been well explored in relation to birth, partly because of the impoverished theoretical frame-works often guiding research. While some feminist researchers have recently moved towards Foucauldian approaches (see Simonds, 2002; Maher, 2003; Martin, 2003; Chadwick & Foster, 2013), birth scholarship and feminist politics often remain caught in frameworks that define agency and choice in narrow, disembodied and neoliberal terms. In this book, power will be understood (following Foucault) as productive, embodied, relational, capillary-like and intertwined with modes of resistance (Sawicki, 1991; Faith, 1994; Root & Browner, 2001). As such, women's birth narratives will be read as embedded and entangled with/in discursive and soci-omaterial relations of power. Birth is an event that always involves multiple modes of power and politics. While biomedicalization remains a central (globally signifi-cant) force shaping the ways in which women give birth, it is always articulated in relation to other modes of power, politics and sociomaterialities. As this book will show, 'biomedicalization' is not a singular or universal process. 'Other' modes of power have been largely neglected in the social science and feminist literature on birth, including gender, race, class and coloniality. Critically, this book shows that these modes of power are not separate or discrete but are themselves "relational materialities" (Fox & Alldred, 2017, p. 27) that mingle, intersect and intra-act.

While a Foucauldian approach to bodies and power is central to this book, it is supplemented by other theories. Exploring the corporeal politics of birth requires a hybrid theoretical approach capable of thinking through the intra-relations between fleshy embodied experience, sociomaterialities and discourse. While Foucauldian approaches emphasize the intertwined dynamic between power/resistance, and the subject is theoretically cast as, "a resisting and active subject, as well as a disciplined and normalized subject" (McLaren, 2002, p. 59), in practice most Foucauldian studies do not engage with the possibility that sensual, embodied, affective and fleshy forces and energies might exceed and disrupt the parameters of discourse and disciplinary modes of power. Instead, power and discourse are often assumed to produce interiority (see McLaren, 2002), and there is little recognition that tactile bodily and material forces might have agency or affective energies of their own. Foucault himself was interested in the ways in which the material-discursive might exceed or leak beyond language and words. As he notes,

> Of course, discourses are composed of signs but what they do is more than use these signs to designate things. It is this *more* that renders them irreducible to language (*langue*) and to speech. It is this 'more' that we must reveal and describe.
>
> *(Foucault, 1972, p. 49; emphasis in original)*

Ironically, in order to explore these issues further, it is necessary to look to other theoretical conceptualizations of bodies and materiality. While Foucault's work might be less 'discourse determinist' than is commonly believed (Hekman, 2010), his work has become commonly associated with the concept of 'body-power' or 'docile bodies.' The resistant body or 'body-resistance,' while an important element of his work, has not been as fully developed. As such, I agree with Crossley (1996) that the Foucauldian concept of 'body-power' needs to be used in conjunction with other theories of the body if we are to grasp the complexities and paradoxes of embodied lives.

New materialism

In order to think the relations between bodies, materiality and discourse beyond a privileging of the linguistic, constructionist theories have developed in new directions. In particular, new materialist theory has emerged as a result of frustrations with the 'discourse determinism' of constructionism. New materialism does not reject the insights of constructionism but acknowledges and builds on them

(Hekman, 2010; Frost, 2011; Fox & Alldred, 2017). As a result, new materialists affirm the constitutive power of language and discourse but argue that, "language has been granted too much power" (Barad, 2007, p. 132). To rectify this, the constitutive and agentic powers of matter, bodies, biology, organisms and the non-human are highlighted (Fausto-Sterling, 2005; Barad, 2007; Bennett, 2010; Frost, 2011). New materialism is a complex, eclectic and interdisciplinary set of ideas with diverse roots in the philosophy of science, feminist theory, poststructuralism, quantum physics, science and technology studies and queer theory. It includes a wide-ranging body of work on assemblage (Deleuze & Guattari, 1987; DeLanda, 2006; Müller, 2015), the post-human (Braidotti, 2013), actor-network theory (Latour, 2005; Müller, 2015) and agential realism (Barad, 2007). Uniting these diverse concepts and theories is the desire to theorize materiality, social life and bodies beyond the confines of discourse, taking into account the agency and relationalities of the non-human, machines, things, biology, matter and bodily energies or 'affects.' New materialism thus moves beyond a narrow focus on (human) bodies as discrete objects of inquiry. Bodies are understood as emergent and fluid entities materializing in relation to a wide range of forces, including physiology, sociomateriality, discourse, machines, institutions, matter, objects and ecosystems. In this book, I will be drawing on concepts embedded in new materialist frameworks. While a focus on the physiological dimensions of birthing bodies is beyond the scope of this book and would require different kinds of 'data,' new materialist concepts of assemblage, diffraction and intra-action inform my analytic approach. I briefly outline these concepts below.

Assemblage

The notion of assemblage is drawn from the work of Deleuze and Guattari (1987) and is a key concept in new materialism. An assemblage is defined as, "a multiplicity which is made up of many heterogeneous terms and which establishes liaisons, relations between them" (Deleuze & Parnet, 1987, p. 69). Assemblages can be thought of as emergent and relational networks, which include a wide variety of heterogeneous elements and forces, including: machines, discourses, architectures, animal and human bodies, biologies, norms, histories, technologies, institutions and materialities. These merge and collide in potentially unexpected directions, creating new entities and outcomes. As noted by Fox and Alldred (2015, p. 401), the heterogeneous elements that comprise particular assemblages materialize in, "unpredictable ways around actions and events" (Fox & Alldred, 2015, p. 401). Assemblages are relational arrangements that are not fixed or pre-determined. According to Müller (2015) assemblages are *sociomaterial* and non-dualist, disrupting any clear divide between nature and culture, social and individual, language and matter, bodies and politics. Things, bodies, selves and discourses are seen as having no fixed or essential ontological status but become meaningful—or materialize— only in relation to other things, bodies, selves, discourses and materialities. Agency is rethought as a product of particular assemblages, troubling the notion that agency is something that an individual self or subject 'has' or 'exerts.' As a result, agency is seen as a capacity generated in assemblages. It is not intrinsic to human selves or a product of (human) discourse. Instead, non-human animals, machines, organisms, genes, environments, discourses, hormones and other forms and forces of matter are all imbued with agency, power and capacities that materialize in particular assemblages. Assemblages are regarded as performative and productive, comprised of relational exchanges that result in unpredictable affective flows and the generation of capacities, agencies, embodied subjects and ontologies.

In new materialist thinking, assemblages are thus seen, not as static arrangements of elements, objects, bodies and things, but as dynamic and unpredictable flows of intensities and energies moving between, within and among constituent parts. The various things, bodies, machines, norms, identities and discourses involved in an assemblage do not merely interact (thereby assuming some static separation between constituent elements); they *intra-act*. The introduction of the idea of intra-action (rather than interaction) is an important move. It troubles the idea that there are pre-existing, coherent things, bodies and categories and insists that things, meanings, selves, identities and bodies materialize with/in relations of heterogeneity in particular assemblages. The focus shifts from the ways in which (stable, coherent) differences 'interact' to looking at *practices of differings*. In the collision/s between parts, things, forces, words, bodies and energies, new relations and configurations are produced and heterogeneous terms and elements are remade. While Barad (2007) refers to concepts of 'intra-action' and 'entanglement' to capture these dynamics, a similar notion of the 'mangle' was introduced by Pickering (1995) and elaborated by Hekman (2010). Mangles are 'impure' and messy networks in which things, machines, discourses and other elements, are 'mixed up' to produce unpredictable and diverse outcomes (Hekman, 2010). The concepts of intra-action, entanglements and mangles allow for a non-essentialist approach to birth that focuses on processes, practices, enactments and becomings. No neat separation can be upheld between constituent parts of an assemblage; instead, they merge, blur, collide and form patterns of organization, arrangement and difference depending on diffracting relations and "interference patterns" (Haraway, 1997, p. 16). According to new materialism, differences such as race, class, gender, disability and sexuality are not coherent or static categories that exist independently or 'intersect.' Instead, they are entangled and relational phenomena that materialize in particular assemblages.

As a result, some have argued that assemblage is a more productive concept than intersectionality (Puar, 2007, 2012; Geerts & Van der Tuin, 2013). While intersectionality claims to resist 'single-axis thinking' and aims to explore the complex interaction of multiple axes of difference (see Collins & Bilge, 2016), the framework arguably remains mired by categorical and essentialist thinking and a tendency to see differences as stable entities. Puar (2012, p. 56) argues that intersectional approaches, "fail to account for the mutual constitution and indeterminacy of gender, sexuality, race, class and nation." Theorists have also critiqued the limited conceptualization of power that frames intersectionality theory. According to

Geerts and Van der Tuin (2013), intersectionality is limited by its conception of power as only repressive and oppressive and lacks the ability to theorize or analyze the complexities of agency and resistance. Assemblage is regarded as a more productive concept because it shifts the focus away from categories and the assumption that axes of difference are stable components, to processes of materialization, diffraction and becoming (Puar, 2007).

Drawing on the new materialist concept of assemblage means the rejection of birth as a stable, decontextualized, biological event that is separate from culture and politics. Instead, birth is reconceived as a series of enactments or an emergent assemblage involving heterogeneous forces, relations and components. As will be shown in this book, birth is never singular but materializes in relation to intra-acting sociomaterialities and ontological politics. Stories about birth can also be thought of as assemblages. While stories would typically be regarded in constructionism as belonging to the realm of words, language and discourse, new materialist approaches allow stories to be reconceptualized as material-discursive assemblages through which bodies, boundaries, capacities and subjectivities are (partially) constituted. Birth stories are thus not reflections of 'what really happened' or pure products of discourse that bare a tenuous relationship to events. Instead, they are themselves material enactments, infused with 'patterns of interference' (Haraway, 1997) based on the overlap between heterogeneous elements, including fleshy bodies, discourse, norms and relational flows. Birth stories thus tell of particular birth assemblages or 'event-assemblages' (Fox & Alldred, 2017), acting as reconfigurations, diffractions and performances of these events. Furthermore, the telling and performance of birth stories, as part of the research process, can also be thought of as a sociomaterial assemblage. Fox and Alldred (2017) distinguish between 'research-assemblages' and 'event-assemblages' to think the dynamics between the event being explored and the research process. As opposed to a constructionist view, which often regards research findings as sociohistorical or discursive products that have a tenuous relationship to events and experiences or as constitutive of the objects/events being explored, new materialist analyses regard 'research-assemblages' and 'event-assemblages' as relational entanglements. In this book, birth stories will be regarded as sociomaterial entanglements of fleshy, embodied enactments, involving, "patterns of difference that make a difference" (Barad, 2007, p. 72).

Onto-epistemology

New materialism involves a shift from questions of epistemology to ontology. Theorists focus on the nature of things, matter and modes of being rather than questions of how to gain legitimate knowledge of the world (Fox & Alldred, 2017). As a result, the focus moves from questions about representation to ontological politics (Mol, 2002). Relational and entangled discursive and sociomaterial enactments literally make and materialize worlds, realities, bodies and subjectivities. Ontologies are thus conceptualized as fundamentally fluid, shifting, embodied and relational rather than fixed or transcendent (Hekman, 2010). Constructionism, which conceptualizes epistemology and ontology as separate, is characterized by new materialists as stuck within binary or dualist modes of thinking and governed by an underlying logic of separation (Barad, 2007; Van der Tuin, 2014). In Barad's agential realism, which she describes as 'onto-epistemology,' there is no absolute separation between things and words, selves and social life, matter and discourse, human and animal, epistemology or ontology. Entities and things have no predetermined or inherent ontological status. The primary units of analysis are not things or words but entanglements, material-discursive enactments or assemblages made up of 'intra-actions' between heterogeneous elements. It is through these intra-actions that boundaries, meanings, bodies, affective flows, agency, subjectivities and fluid ontologies are established (Barad, 2007).

New materialist analysis is regarded as 'posthuman,' displacing individual human selves as sources of knowledge and agency. From a focus on individual human subjects, agency and identity politics, or the power of the discursive, the focus shifts to relational becomings and concepts of assemblage, entanglement and intra-action. Questions shift from the relationship between bodies, things and words to, "matters of practices, doings and actions" (Barad, 2007, p. 135). Words do not reflect preexisting things nor do they determine the world. Materiality and discourse are regarded as entangled, with discursive practices regarded, "not as human-based activities but specific material (re)configurings of the world through which boundaries, properties, and meanings are differentially enacted" (p. 183). While poststructuralist theorists such as Butler (1993) claim that bodies materialize as effects of discursive and social forces, new materialist theory argues that the forces at play in the materialization of bodies are not only sociodiscursive and that not only human bodies are produced (Barad, 2007). Assumed and accepted boundaries between bodies and language are troubled. Instead of being a blank template awaiting inscription and discursive materialization, the body is seen as, "an agential reality with its own causal role in making meaning" (Hames-Garcia, 2008, p. 327). In new materialism, bodies are fleshy physiologies that become-in-relation, have agential power and carry traces of historical and ideological diffractions in their bones, flesh, speech, practices and corporeal way of being in the world (Hames-Garcia, 2008).

Diffraction

Diffraction is a concept used by new materialist thinkers (Haraway, 1997; Barad, 2007; Van der Tuin, 2014) as a metaphor for an alternative understanding of the world. Barad (2007) describes diffraction as, "patterns of difference that make a difference" (p. 72) and argues that diffraction demonstrates, "the entangled structure of the changing and contingent ontology of the world" (p. 73). A concept drawn from physics, diffraction describes the physical phenomenon of patterns, combinations and interferences that occur when waves overlap and the ways in which waves bend, ripple, swirl or radiate upon encountering an obstacle (Barad, 2007). Diffractive approaches are interested in exploring the dynamic and performative effects (and affects) produced by intra-acting differences. According to Van der Tuin (2014), the goal is to use diffraction as a conceptual tool to show differences *differing*. In line with a diffractive approach, the embodied subject can be recon-ceptualized as a diffractive sociomaterial movement or ripple of voices, histories, ideologies and fleshy and physiological energies. While diffraction becomes an object of study and theoretical lens, it is also a methodological approach, critical praxis and way of reading (Barad, 2007; Van der Tuin, 2014). Theories and con-cepts are read through one another and there is no privileging of one particular 'discipline' or tradition. A diffractive approach, "does not take separateness to be an inherent feature of how the world is" (p. 136). Ontology, epistemology and ethics are not regarded as separate. Practices of research are seen as ethical engagements that *matter*. According to Barad (2007, p. 91), "making knowledge is not simply about making facts but about making worlds."

In this book, women's birth narratives will be read diffractively as entangle-ments and multiple *relatings*. These narratives will not be seen as 'just words,' with the authentic real, fleshy and material situated somewhere elsewhere but will be regarded as material-discursive practices or "dynamic topological reconfigurings/ entanglements/relationalities" (Barad, 2007, p. 141). Birth stories will be shown to be heterogeneous and performative events in which multiple ideologies, dis-courses, norms, histories and materialities diffractively ripple, overlap and swirl. Birthing bodies will be conceptualized as points of diffraction (collision points) between multiplicities of entanglements. Bodies are inscribed, not by coherent, pre-determined meanings or fixed discourses, but by interference patterns created by entangled diffractions in particular material-discursive ensembles (Haraway, 1997). At the same time, they are part of these diffraction patterns and themselves exert agential power in relation to other forces/entities in particular assemblages. As such they are always plural becomings, carrying and incorporating residues of multiple entangled relatings and interference patterns and yet are also agentic with material capacities and the power to affect. In line with a diffractive methodology, the point of analysis shifts from describing or replicating to "a mapping of interfer-ence" (Haraway, 1992, p. 300).

But how do we map interference points or diffraction patterns in qualitative analysis? And how do we deal with the tensions involved in trying to apply a *sociomaterial* analysis to birth narratives? While new materialists reject the separation between language and materiality as false and focus on enactments and practices as points of analysis, the exact relations between language, discourse and bodies are not always well explicated beyond the notion of 'entanglements.' For the purposes of this project, which deals with birth narratives as the central source of 'data,' it is critical to explore how storytelling about birth can be analyzed diffractively and as sociomaterial practices. To do so means asking questions about the entangled relations between bodies and language, narrative and ideology and storytelling and politics. To this end, I draw on the work of Julia Kristeva as a frame for theorizing the materiality of language and developing an understanding of bodies, narratives and selves as collision points made up of multiple, disruptive and diffracting voices.

Kristeva and the materiality of language: reading diffractively

Julia Kristeva's work provides a useful frame for thinking about the entanglements between corporeality and discourse that radically destabilizes the separation between language and the body. Her notion of the 'speaking body' troubles assumptions of bodies as mute, passive and somehow outside language *and* highlights the embodied, material and fleshy nature of language itself. In her account, language is not a disembodied transcendent force but operates in, through and on fleshy bodies. Furthermore, language is not just spoken *by* bodies but is thoroughly enfleshed, with meaning-making itself dependent on fleshy energies. Kristeva theorizes the embodied subject as "a strange fold" situated like "an intersection or crossroads" between the practices of culture, discourse, the body and ideology (Boulous-Walker, 1998, p. 105) and offers a complex theorization of the fleshiness of language. In her formulation, language does not just refer to a formal system of words, linguistic structures, meanings and discourses. Language is a signifying embodied process in which both bodily energies and sociomaterialities become transfused (Chadwick, 2017a). Kristeva departs from other poststructuralists by arguing that language cannot be approached or understood apart from 'the speaking being' or embodied subject whose "living energy transfuses meaning into language" (p. 59). The speaking body is brought back into language and language is reconceptualized as an entanglement between flesh, ideology and sociocultural dynamics.

In her work, Kristeva prefers to speak of the 'signifying process' rather than language or discourse. This process is made up of two different orders, namely: a semiotic and symbolic mode, both of which are necessary for making meaning and making subjects (Kristeva, 1984). The symbolic is defined as, "clear and orderly meaning" (McAfee, 2004, p. 15), referring to the grammar, syntax and logic of language. The semiotic evades easy definition. According to Grosz (1989, p. 43), the semiotic is, "the energies, rhythms, forces and corporeal residues necessary for representation." Bodily and physiological energies are conceptualized as an integral part of language. The semiotic, as bodily, vocal and fleshy rhythms, sensual and affective residues, mingles and morphs with/through symbolic language and material-discursive ensembles (or assemblages). Fleshy energies breathe living energy into language and convert static words into a sensual and embodied matrix of meaning. The semiotic mode is also a constant source of disruption and interruption, which can be thought through the new materialist concept of diffraction in which "interference patterns" (Haraway, 1997) constantly threaten to destabilize coherence, univocality, sameness and homogeneity (Boulous-Walker, 1998). Language and bodies are entangled and mutually infiltrated and colonized—there are no stable boundary lines. As a result, embodied selves, caught in a messy 'mangle' of relations (Hekman, 2010) are constantly in a state of contradiction and disruption. As in the new materialism, 'the body' and its fleshy materiality are not conceptualized as separate from language and discourse but as complexly entangled. The embodied subject is a field of contradiction, disruption and diffraction—there is no univocal, stable or singular self. Kristeva also argues that language itself materializes in relation to material energies that are enfleshed and diffracted in/through the sociocultural. Moreover, the Symbolic, "the social realm" (Oliver, 1993, p. 10) is also inscribed within the matter of bodies and flesh; thus, "the dynamics that operate the Symbolic are already working within the material of the body" (p. 3). Like Donna Haraway, a key figure in 'new materialism,' Kristeva emphasizes the instability of boundaries defining bodies, culture, language and subjects.

Similarly to new materialist thinkers, Kristeva (1980, 1984, 1986a) conceptualizes subjects, bodies and discourse as moving and emergent processes. Subjectivity is regarded, not as an essence or a discursive effect, but as a dialectical movement or becoming. The Kristevan subject is always 'in process' and never finalized. Kristeva, however, goes beyond new materialism in offering a nuanced theory explicating the ways in which fleshy materialities infuse, interrupt, enable and infiltrate language. Language itself is seen as fractured, relational, corpomaterial and spoken by/through fleshy bodies. As a result, the speaking being is regarded as central to theorizing the entanglements between language and materiality. Kristeva conceptualizes language, not as representative or constructive, but as corporeal, enfleshed and itself a site/point of diffraction, heterogeneity and disruption. New materialists, on the other hand, often eschew discussions about language and prefer to talk of discursive practices (Barad, 2007). According to Barad (2007, p. 149), discursive practices are, "not speech acts, linguistic representations or even linguistic performances." Moreover, they are not human-based activities. Language, words and representations are often regarded dismissively. For example, Barad (2007, p. 146) refers pejoratively to, "mere spoken or written words." Barad also singles out language as that which has been, "granted too much power" (p. 132). The decentering of language in new materialism is a response to the emphasis on the linguistic, representation and discourse in poststructuralism. As a result, language itself has been undertheorized in new materialism, particularly in relation to its forceful corpomateriality. I agree with MacLure (2013, p. 663) that "there is more work to be done on the status of language itself within a materialist research practice." Language can no longer be expected to "work in the old ways" (p. 663) of poststructuralism and discourse theory but needs radical rethinking. MacLure (2013) calls for approaches that are able to engage with the complex materiality of language—"the fact that language is in and of the body; always issuing from the body; being impeded by the body; affecting other bodies" (p. 663). Kristeva's theory offers a productive framework with which to begin this work. Her work also retains an engagement with 'the speaking being' that is often missing from both poststructuralist and new materialist work. As a result, embodied subjects run the risk of disappearing in both theoretical schools.

In this book, acts of storytelling are regarded as fleshy and sociomaterial performances. In line with an approach that draws on new materialism and Kristevan theory, acts of telling are seen as embodied and emergent enactments. They are also sociomaterial assemblages made up of a swirling and moving mix of fleshy intra-actions, affective residues, diffracting voices (ideological, institutional, discursive and moral), socioeconomics, norms and sociocultural narrative frames. They (re)enact the birth event in pulsating and crackling acts of telling. They also materialize birth in relation to the sociorelational and material dynamics of the narrative encounter. Thinking Kristeva's theory of the fleshy, linguistic and performative 'subject-in-process' with new materialist concepts, opens productive analytic and methodological spaces for the exploration of fleshy acts of telling and diffractive 'patterns of interference' (Haraway, 1997). I now turn to methodological issues and ask how best to utilize the theoretical concepts already outlined in analytic work. I explore the methodological implications of engaging in a "mapping of interference" (Haraway, 1992, p. 300), arguing that a dialogical narrative approach is well suited to the aims of diffractive analysis.

Methodological diffractions: tracing disruptive voices

What methodological tools are needed to trace 'patterns of interference' (Haraway, 1997) or the heterogeneous play of voices, differings and fleshy energies in birth storytelling? The usual methods (i.e. thematic analysis, discourse analysis) will not suffice. Most qualitative analytic methods are geared towards lumping data into 'themes' and producing codes and categories or 'patterns of sameness.' Contradictions, discontinuities and hermeneutical interruptions are often regarded as things to be 'smoothed over' and 'ironed out' of analysis. If we are to take disruption seriously in analysis, we must guard against pruning the embodied excesses of speech out of transcriptions. Taking the corpomateriality of language seriously means tending carefully to practices of transcription—a 'critical moment' in the research process in which embodied voices are often muted and lost.

My approach to transcription in this project was thus geared towards preserving, as far as possible, the fleshy vocal energies of acts of telling and "talk as a vital performative element of meaning-making" (Chadwick, 2017a, p. 61). Respecting fleshy tellings is not just about the use of notation and codes to denote the bodily dimensions of speech (which will always falter and fall short). It is also about the ways in which speech and utterances are represented on the page. My approach was thus framed by Kristevan theory and by what has been termed the 'ethnopoetic' style of transcription in which the poetic and performative aspects of storytelling are highlighted (see Blommaert, 2006). Ethnopoetic transcription is interested in representing the performative qualities of talk and telling and encourages the reader/audience to enter into 're-enactment' of the original telling. The transcription becomes a "sensory experience" and "prompts new forms of performativity from the bodies of the transcript's reader" (O'Dell & Willim, 2013, p. 318). The way words and utterances are arranged on the page is not neutral or insignificant but can function as itself a way of affecting mood and re-performing the rhythm and idiosyncratic flow of a particular narrative (O'Dell & Willim, 2013). Transcripts are sensory texts and echoes and their "rhetorical architecture" (Moore, 2013, p. 15) is an important element in interpretation. The rhythms, vocal peculiarities and idiosyncratic 'ways of telling' that materialize during storytelling are themselves layers of meaning that intra-act with words and formal symbolic language. In ethnopoetics, narratives are conceptualized as performances organized in relation to aesthetic and poetic vocal patterns and not in terms of content (Blommaert, 2006). Thus, critically, "what there is to be told emerges out of how it is being told" (p. 182). *Ways of telling* are analytically important. In this book, I use narrative poems as representational and analytic devices to highlight the performative aspects of storytelling and the excessive and multivocal qualities of telling (see Chapters 6 and 7). These poems offer a way of representing acts of telling as fluid, fleshy and emergent movements involving contradictory, diffractive and heterogeneous embodied voices. Furthermore, they enact transcribed extracts as open and performative texts rather than closed and static empirical reflections of a singular reality.

In Kristevan theory, the semiotic mode of bodily energies and rhythms is a constituent element of meaning-making. The sociomaterial and corporeal are already circulating in/through/as words spoken by embodied subjects. Words alone do not make meaning. This book will show that women's birth stories pulsate with a sense of corporeality, fleshiness and sociomateriality that operates as, "the potentially disruptive meaning that is not quite a meaning below the text" (McAfee, 2004, p. 24) erupting in storytelling as rhyme, repetition, undecipherable utterances, intonation, breath, rhythm, absences and contradictions. Trying to respect and re-enact the bodily energies in transcript texts is challenging and any effort to do so remains interpretive and constructive and does not reflect the final or 'authentic' reality of actual speech acts. All acts of transcription, listening and interpreting are "further sets of transformations in a chain" (Ashmore, Macmillan & Brown, 2004, p. 371). The question, however, remains: how do we listen analytically for the multiple bodies and diffracting, disruptive voices in stories? What modes of qualitative analysis enable engagement with discontinuities, absences, polyvocality and hermeneutical disruptions?

Dialogical modes of narrative analysis, which argue that any one voice is the site of multiple voices (Frank, 2005), is used to frame my analysis in this book. In dialogical narrative analysis, stories are not seen as univocal reflections of experience and the narrator is not regarded as the author or origin-point of the story being told. Stories are heterogenous assemblages told/by through narrators that escape, seep and leak. Dialogical approaches, which respect plurality and non-finalizability as ethical and ontological features of narratives (and narrators), resonate productively with new materialist theories. According to Frank (2010, p. 42), stories are "material semiotic companions" that are comprised of signs but that also *do* things; they "perform themselves through us" (Law, 2000, p. 28) and take material forms (i.e. machines, bodies, objects). Furthermore, storytelling "materializes the semiotic" (Frank, 2010, p. 44). Through words, voice, gestures and breath, the body of the storyteller (re)performs the bodies in and of the story so that what happened or what was imagined can re-materialize in narrative form (Frank, 2010). In commonsense and representationist thinking, experiences happen first and stories are told afterwards. Stories are thus predominantly understood as representations, facsimiles or reflections of what happened. Some narrative scholars have troubled this assumption, arguing that stories do not only happen *after* experiences but that we have experiences only because of particular stories and narrative forms (Frank, 2010). Circulating cultural and local stories thus shape experiences and actions. In relation to birth, this means that women go into the birth event carrying an assorted collection of stories and story fragments which impact on and contributes to shaping their birth experiences. Sociocultural meanings and interpretive frames 'always already' infiltrate enactments of birth.

Bodies tell and perform stories. Stories are entanglements of fleshy, sensory experiences, socially accepted narrative forms/genres and sociomaterialities. Circulating in/through stories are also modes of disruption and interference in the form of moral, sociomaterial and ideological interpellations. These interpellations emerge in and through stories as diffractive resonances or voices that materialize in acts of telling. Stories thus resound with heterogenous voices and can be thought of as "textures of resonances" (Frank, 2010, p. 37). The body tells stories via words, plot lines and genres but the body also speaks through stories in other, irreducible ways and with other (sometimes contradictory) meanings (breath, tone, gesture, laughter, inarticulate sounds, rhythm and intonation). As pointed out by Frank (1995, p. 2), "hearing traces of the body in the story is not easy" and requires a different level of analytic listening.

This book will show that it is not just the sensual, fleshy body that speaks through stories. Ideologies and sociomaterialities also speak. Bodies, ideologies and sociomaterialities can be usefully thought of as 'disruptive voices,' which challenge and counter narrative order, univocality and homogeneity. The idea of 'disruptive voices' will be shown to be analytically useful in subsequent analytic chapters. For example, a focus on stories as assemblages of *differing voices* (including ideological, moral, fleshy and sociomaterial voices) that disrupt singularity and homogeneity opens up spaces to begin to think about engaging with the idea of diffraction in analysis. The jostling and polyphonic voices in stories can be thought of as interruptions or 'patterns of interference' (Haraway, 1997). Any individual story is an emergent performance and site of multiple intra-acting sociomaterialities, stories and ideological forces. Sociomaterialities thus emerge as disruptive, diffracting and interrupting voices that shape, produce and colonize acts of telling.

Materialist feminist approaches have long conceptualized contradictions, gaps and disruptions within texts as refractions of sociomaterial and structural conditions (see Hennessey, 1993; Ebert, 1996; Boulous-Walker, 1998). According to Ebert (1996, p. 7), ideology critique is, "a mode of knowing that inquires into what is not said, into the silences and the suppressed or missing" with the aim of exploring power and socioeconomic relations. Althusser's notion of ideological 'interpellation' also resonates productively with the concept of diffraction, enabling an understanding of the ways in which subjects are positioned by, and caught between, multiple ideological voices (see Van der Tuin, 2014). In Althusser's conceptualization, interpellation refers to the process whereby subjects recognize themselves and are positioned (as particular kinds of selves) in relation to ideologies via discursive and sociomaterial acts of 'hailing.' As such, interpellation is a process whereby both selves and ideologies become or materialize. Interpellations thus act as potential modes of interference and disturbance. Furthermore, interpellation is not only linguistic but is also sociomaterial—for example, the arrangement of objects and machines in a labor ward 'hails' particular actions, affects and forms of being from birthing women (i.e. acting as a patient and medical object). Interpellative disruptions are also not singular affairs but are always comprised of plural, contradictory and heterogeneous voices and disturbances (Van der Tuin, 2014) that materialize with/in and in relation to material-discursive ensembles or 'assemblages.'

While Frank's (2005) dialogical approach to narrative analysis sets out five 'commitments' of the method, not a lot of detail is provided about how to go about *doing* a dialogical narrative analysis. This is where analytic tools developed in the Listening Guide (see Gilligan et al., 2003) prove to be useful. The Listening Guide is a variant of narrative analysis developed by Carol Gilligan and colleagues in the 1980s. This method is fundamentally dialogical in its analytic strategies and understands selves as composites of multiple and potentially contradictory (what is termed 'contrapuntal') voices. Narratives are thus conceptualized as made up of multiple voices, echoes and resonances. While the method is rooted in realist onto-epistemology, the strategies and analytic tools it provides can be productively utilized when read through other theoretical lenses. Most importantly, the proposed use of 'I poems' as analytic strategy to trace the shifting movement of the 'I voice' in/through storytelling is an important listening and analytic device. The analyst highlights the use of the 'I pronoun' and associated words/phrases throughout the narrative and then constructs an 'I poem' by placing each phrase on a separate line. A poetic representation of the moving 'I voice' of the narrator is thus assembled, allowing for a different way of listening to the narrator and of discerning the multiple voices that resonate or echo within any one narrative. In my own use of the Listening Guide (see Chadwick, 2009, 2012, 2017a), I have played with a variety of 'pronoun poems' including tracing the use of 'they,' 'we' and 'it' in addition to the 'I' voice. While not advocated as a part of the Listening Guide method, representing stories in poetic form has several advantages over the traditional use of blocks of quoted extracts. It re-engages, affirms and highlights the performative and dialogical qualities of telling stories (and transcribing them) as opposed to muting these aspects by representing them in decontextualized and abbreviated chunks. It also allows the moving play of differing, multiple and contrapuntal voices to be traced and represented within individual stories.

A brief outline of the book

Over the course of this book, I explore the ways in which birthing bodies emerge *as multiple*. I trouble the notion that there is any singular birthing body and explore the heterogeneous enactments of birthing corporeality within and across sociomaterial relations of *differings*. In addition to exploring the birthing body as multiple, I also highlight the multivocality of birth stories as they were told across race/class divides. I highlight everyday enactments of embodied inequality as played out in women's birth narratives and trace the 'ontological politics' (Mol, 2002) framing and vitalizing these inequalities.

Chapter 2 begins by engaging with the 'politics of framing.' This chapter explores the ways in which birthing bodies have been framed and enacted in biomedicine, psychological research, global activism and feminist politics. I argue that engagement with the fleshy corporeality of birth has largely been missing from the social science literature and activist agendas. At the same time, however, assumptions about the ontologies of birthing bodies pervade research, biomedicine and birth politics. In this chapter, I explore these assumptions, arguing that dualist frames and racist colonial logic continues to shape the ways we think about birth.

My analysis of birthing bodies as multiplicities enacted and diffracted through women's birth stories is presented over the course of four chapters (see Chapters 3–6). Chapter 3 focuses on the ways biomedical ontologies of power materialized as narrative scripts in women's stories. This chapter shows how 'clockwork birth' emerged as a central mode of narrative storytelling. This script was biomedically derived and framed both privileged and low-income women's birth experiences and stories. However, the diffractive enactments of 'clockwork bodies' as biomedical entities differed according to sociomateriality, resulting in the materialization of different kinds of biomedical bodies in particular settings. Biomedical power is shown in this chapter to be thoroughly entangled with/in women's narratives and their sociomaterial and fleshy experiences of birth, at times enabling embodied forms of agency and at others working to discipline bodies and mute the psychofleshy birth experience.

Chapter 4 focuses on 'risky bodies' as enacted in women's birth stories. This chapter extends the analysis of biomedical power started in Chapter 3 by exploring the different 'risk economies' materializing in women's birth narratives. I show that the politics of risk is fundamentally entangled with sociomaterial locations, with very different biomedical risk economies emerging in the stories of privileged and low-income women. Thus, while biomedical risk was enacted via heightened visibility and surveillance in the private sector, in the public sector women were often subject to biomedical *invisibilization*. This chapter also shows that women enacted multiple forms of risk in their stories. The 'risky body' of birth was not singular and risk, in relation to birth, was not only about biomedical risk. Women were thus worried about other risks, including the distinctive corporeal risks of the laboring/ birthing body (i.e. loss of dignity and exposure). In the public sector, women also negotiated the risks of dehumanization, violence and the absence of medical care.

Chapter 5 explores the violations produced in birth narratives. In particular, I focus on the 'gentle violences' materializing in/through women's tellings. This chapter thus 'looks sideways' (Žižek, 2008) and focuses on the normalized and often hidden forms of violence that are enacted during labor/birth. I show how 'gentle violence,' embedded in the norms, sociomaterial and affective currents of assemblages, work to generate passive subjectivities, constricted forms of agency and docile bodies, particularly in public sector contexts. Embodied oppressions, including constraints on embodied agency, shaming, violations of dignity, structural disrespect and the denial of embodied personhood, were also reproduced as 'normal' within particular birth assemblages.

While Chapters 3–5 focus on the ways in which normative relations of power were interwoven with women's experiences, choices and narratives of birth, Chapter 6 looks at the other side of power—namely: subversion, resistance and countering. In this chapter, I look at the ways in which birth stories exceeded, leaked and 'spoke back' against normative relations of power. This chapter adopts a creative analytic approach fusing dialogical narrative analysis (Frank, 2010) with poetic representational devices (Gilligan et al., 2003) to explore the contradictions, multiplicities and excessive qualities of birth storytelling. I argue that fleshy bodies are key to hearing moments of resistance and focus particularly on the bodily *excess* in storytelling. I show how comedy and humor functioned as modes of embodied resistance that mocked normative narratives and subverted the logic and assumptions of dominant storylines of birth. I also show how subversion operated in/through the telling of the psychofleshy labor/birth experience. Through fleshy eruptions, birthing bodies *spoke back* against erasure, telling pleasure and distress as embodied enactments. Lastly, in this chapter I also show how some low-income women enacted 'loud' forms of resistance by telling testimonies of violation that enabled them to reflexively enact agency (through storytelling) and take a stand against birthing injustices.

Chapters 7 and 8 conclude the book by asking—what *matters* in relation to birth? How can we move birth politics beyond dualist frames and problematic idealizations and valorizations? In order to explore this question, I focus on what matters to women by exploring how they articulate and enact *feelings* about their birth experiences. To this end, I present a 'collective assemblage of voices' drawn from women's narratives and use this multivocal weave to explore what matters in relation to birth. I argue that birthing bodies matter and that the feelings women have about their births reveal important insights into the sociomaterial and ontological relations that frame birth in particular assemblages. I conclude that vitalizing birth politics requires the development of alternative ontologies of birth that valorize embodied ethicality and recognize embodied personhood.

2

BIRTHING BODIES

The politics of framing

Birth has been extensively researched since the 1970s, with a wide-range of literature published in sociology, history, nursing, anthropology, psychology and public health. Various topics have been explored, including: risk and birth, factors associated with 'birth satisfaction,' medicalization, choice and control, social support, intersectional issues and implications of mode and place of birth. Women's experiences of birth have been widely documented, particularly in Euro-American settings. Despite this extensive engagement, little attention has been paid to the embodied or corporeal aspects of birth. This is surprising considering that birth is a powerful bodily event (Walsh, 2010) and given the broader 'turn to bodies' in the social sciences from the 1980s onwards (Turner, 1984; Frank, 1990; Shilling, 1993). While researchers have largely avoided engaging with birthing bodies, there is a substantial literature on other procreative and reproductive modes of embodiment—i.e. pregnancy (see Lupton, 1999a; Schmied & Lupton, 2001a; Elvey, 2003; Warren & Brewis, 2004; Nash, 2012) and breastfeeding (Blum, 1999; Bartlett, 2002; Hausman, 2007; Boyer, 2012). This makes the silence on birthing bodies even more puzzling.

While explicit engagement with the corporeality of birth has been largely missing, ontological assumptions about birthing bodies nonetheless pervade birth scholarship, everyday birth practices, birth activisms and transnational debates. In this chapter, I explore some of these assumptions, showing that mind–body dualism, nature–culture binaries and residues of colonial and racist thinking, continue to shape the ways we think about birth. These frames are not just abstract representations of birth, but act to materialize and enact birth and birthing bodies in particular ways. As mentioned in Chapter 1, a key focus of this book is the ontological politics of birth. In line with new materialism, ontologies are not fixed or given but are "highly topical matters" (Mol, 2002, p. 7) and everyday enactments that contribute to the materializations of worlds, bodies and realities. As a result, ontological assumptions about birthing bodies—i.e. what they 'are,' what they can do and how to manage, treat and research them—are not just representations, perspectives or forms of knowledge; they are sociomaterial enactments which matter (Mol, 2002). This chapter explores ontological framings of the body that births in biomedicine, psychology, global birth politics and activism. I also briefly outline the small body of qualitative research that has explored aspects of birthing embodiment.

Framing birthing bodies: the biomedical and biological body

The biomedical body is one of the dominant ontologies of the body in modernity (Ettorre, 1998). In biomedical terms, bodies are biological objects rather than embodied subjects and the person in/of the body is regarded as irrelevant to medical practice. Biomedical assumptions about the nature of the body, founded upon Cartesian dualism, are not confined to medical examination rooms, medical experts or hospitals but have become cultural commonsense, framing everyday understandings about what bodies 'are' (Ettorre, 2002). In biomedical terms, the birthing body is a faulty machine or "collection of parts" (Rothman, 1982, p. 35) which biomedicine can fix, improve and manipulate (Martin, 1987; Sbisà, 1996; Davis-Floyd, 2003). Abnormalities are expected during labor/birth, with the parameters of 'normality' becoming ever narrower in biomedical practice (Scamell, 2011). The birthing body is also regarded as a purely physiological entity that operates separately from 'mind,' subjectivity and self. These framings shape the ways women are treated during labor/birth, enacting the birthing body as an object-body to be managed, controlled, measured, probed and regulated. Feelings, environments, wishes, desires and meanings are seen as separate from the physiological workings of the body. Women in the Global North have been found to internalize biomedical vocabularies of the body with images of fragmentation, disembodiment and body/self separation rife in women's talk about their birth experiences (see Martin, 1987; Sbisà, 1996).

The biomedical body, as risky, defective and in need of medical intervention, is a dominant interpretation of the birthing body. While feminist scholars have critiqued medicalized concepts of the birthing body as pathological, they have not always contested the dualisms underpinning these conceptions. Often feminists have focused their attention on the other side of the dualism (i.e. culture and sociality), arguing that birth is a sociocultural event overlaid with multiple meanings, rituals and practices (Jordan, 1993; Michaelson, 1988; Davis-Floyd, 2003). At the same time, birthing bodies have often been left untheorized and dualisms intact. For example, while conceptualizing birth as a social and psychological event, Oakley (1980) nonetheless continues to frame the birthing body as solely a biological entity and foundational template on which socialization acts. Although overlaid by cultural and social meanings, birth is seen in Oakley's research as "a biological event" (Oakley, 1980, p. 7). Feminist anthropologists and sociologists have thus often emphasized the social and cultural aspects of birth but left ontological assumptions about birthing bodies, as primarily (static and bounded) biological entities, uncontested. What feminist scholars have contested are biomedical interpretations of the birthing body as pathological, defective and prone to breakdown. To counter these constructions, feminists have reinterpreted the biological or 'natural' birthing body in positive and empowering ways as powerful, capable and affirming (see Martin, 1987; Macdonald, 2006; Cheyney, 2008).

For many middle-class women, birth choices and sensemaking often revolve around the competing constructs of biomedical or 'natural' birthing bodies (Davis-Floyd, 2003). Both constructs are, however, based on the assumption that the birthing body is essentially a stable biological body. It is either a biological body prone to breakdown and in need of medical intervention or it is a 'natural' body imbued with instinctive power and innate capacities to birth without medicalization. The ontological assumption that birthing bodies are essentially (static, universal and bounded) biological entities thus underpins different approaches to birth, including biomedical and natural birth models. The persistence of the medical–natural birth dichotomy, identified by some birth scholars as an impediment to the development of birth politics and scholarship in new directions (see Walsh, 2010) is, in my view, a product of entrenched dualist assumptions about the body that births.

While doing little to disrupt mind–body, nature–culture, medical–natural and biological–social dualisms, the work done by feminist anthropologists to show that birth is a sociocultural affair has nonetheless been important. Anthropologists such as Robbie Davis-Floyd (2003) have shown that sociocultural myths and rituals pertaining to birth apply not only to 'traditional' cultures, but also to Western societies. Furthermore, Davis-Floyd (1994) has argued that a biomedical or 'technocratic' approach to birth is itself a specific cultural system embedded in Western approaches to knowledge, and that obstetrical procedures function as a series of rituals that reiterate core Western assumptions about bodies, nature, gender and technology. Feminist scholars have also provided strong critiques of the dangers and problems associated with the 'medicalization' of birth and have theorized medicalized birth as a patriarchal ideology (Cahill, 2001). According to Rothman (1982), medicalized birth is underpinned by the 'ideology of technology' in which the unpredictability, inherent pathology and volatility of birthing bodies (as defined by patriarchal medicine) is seen as conquered by obstetric technology and interventions. Despite different materializations depending on local contexts, a biomedical conception of the body that births has global hegemonic status (see Davis-Floyd, 2003). Ironically, while many middle-class women in the Global North are engaged in struggles to 'demedicalize' birth, Johnson (2016) argues that medicalization is not necessarily a problem for disadvantaged women in the North or women located in Southern settings.

At this point it might be useful to pause and ask: *what* medicalization? By 'medicalization' do we mean potentially life-saving technology and interventions or a conceptual and sociomaterial system that brings particular ontologies of birth (and birthing bodies) into being? According to Garry (2001), there is an important difference between medicine and medicalization. Medicalization refers to the process whereby normal life events (i.e. birth and the menopause) become redefined as dysfunctional and unable to proceed without medical intervention or treatment (Purdy, 2001) and has been theorized by feminists as a form of social control. Garry (2001) argues that the feminist critique of medicalization does not automatically mean that medical treatment and intervention is also rejected—i.e. "one can desire medicine without desiring medicalization" (p. 262). A key problem with the feminist critique of biomedical birth has been that medical technology has at times been defined as inherently disempowering and negative (Rothman, 1982; Cahill, 2001). This has entrenched and reiterated dualist thinking in which medicine/nature are conceptualized as binary opposites and reduced birth politics to either/or positionings. In my view, 'medicalization' is a series of ontological framings, enactments and sociomaterial practices in which birthing bodies materialize as medical objects, birth becomes a medical event, technology is valorized over embodied knowledge and the social and personal significance of birth is erased. While the feminist critique of biomedicalized birth has historically been associated with privileged women in Euro-American settings, this has shifted to the point where criticisms of medicalization can no longer be said to only be about privileged women in Northern settings. For example, in Latin America there is a robust and vibrant birth activist movement that is struggling against the medicalization of birth and unnecessary intervention is argued to be a form of 'obstetric violence' (see Pérez D' Gregorio, 2010). Medicalization materializes differently according to geopolitical settings and in relation to bodily differences (class and race). However, resolidifying binary thinking by arguing that medicalization is only a problem for privileged women in the Global North and that marginalized women have no problems with being 'medicalized' during birth (see Johnson, 2016) is not a helpful position for a feminist politics of birth. By reinforcing such dualisms we remain trapped in the endless chain of conceptual binaries that plague birth scholarship. We need to focus instead on mapping and tracing the diffracting ways in which 'medicalization' emerges as a series of ontological and body politics in a range of contexts.

Diffractions

As outlined above, biomedical bodies are biological entities prone to disease and dysfunction that materialize predominantly as objects to be measured, probed and classified by medical experts and technologies (Goldberg, 2002). Furthermore, biomedical ontologies are underpinned by Cartesian dualism in which bodies and minds are regarded as separate entities and bodies are seen as lowly uncivilized matter (Einstein & Shildrick, 2009; Davis & Walker, 2010a). It is important to pause from this compelling yet universalistic tale at this point. We need to ask: does biomedicine operate as a universal system that defines and frames all birthing bodies in the same way? When looking again, and looking diffractively, the answer must be no. Mind–body dualism does not interpellate all bodies in the same way and the biomedical body is not one. Historically, some bodies have been regarded as more lowly, animalistic and uncivilized than others. Scholars of birth and women's health have shown how the denigration of women's bodies is linked to historical ideas about female matter and women's bodily functions as animal-like and repugnant (Moscucci, 1990; Massey, 2005; Ussher, 2006). However, what 'women' are we talking about here? Bodies have never been gendered without at the same time being racialized. According to Lugones (2007), gender and race were fused inextricably in colonial articulations of what it meant to be a human being. Gender was, "thoroughly informed through the coloniality of power" (p. 201), with only white, middle-class women counting as 'proper' women able to access ideals of respectable and civilized femininity. While white women *were* regarded as closer to nature than their white male counterparts, black women (and men) were regarded as savage, animal-like, devoid of civilization and associated with primitive bodily urges. Mind–body dualism is thus not one 'thing' that applies to all human bodies in the same way—instead, as a binary it is thoroughly racialized. This becomes readily apparent when exploring the ways in which birthing bodies have been framed and conceptualized.

From a Euro-American perspective, the birthing body has been predominantly biomedicalized and regarded as a defective machine in need of fixing. As a result, the biomedicalization of birth has been one of the dominant narratives informing feminist scholarship and politics on birth. However, while this narrative is appropriate when thinking about birth in relation to the experiences of white women in the Global North, it simultaneously also erases other narratives that show the entanglements of ideas about birthing bodies, racialization and coloniality. Birthing bodies are not all biomedicalized in the same way. Biomedical conceptions of birthing bodies are entangled with sticky, persistent residues of Eurocentric, colonialist and racist meta-narratives. Processes of racialized othering thus remain important elements of the ontological politics constituting birth. We cannot speak of the biomedicalized birthing body as if it was one thing. Attention must be paid to the differings inherent in the treatment and conceptualization of birthing bodies, both historically and with residues that continue to persist to the present day.

Racialized bodies, 'natural' bodies and colonial appropriations

While birth is widely regarded as a physiological event, the positioning of women in relation to this event differs according to socioeconomics, race, socioculture and geopolitics. Rich, white women have historically been construed as experiencing more pain and difficulty in relation to birth because of their supposedly higher state of civilized femininity. African women, on the other hand, have been cast as more primitive and thus able to give birth painlessly and easily (Cosslett, 1994). The biomedicalization of birth was from the outset a class- and status-related process in which middle- and upper-class European women in the mid-1700s began to display a preference for male birth attendants with their array of instruments (e.g. obstetric forceps) and interventions (Shorter, 1982; Lewis, 1983; Hanson, 2004).

In the 1920s, white middle-class, Euro-American women were again at the fore-front of efforts to access pain-relieving drugs during birth and demanded the right to a pain-free birth experience (Leavitt, 1986; Pollock, 1999). While the bodies of white, privileged Euro-American women were regarded as prone to 'hysterization' (Foucault, 1990) in part because of the supposed clash between civilizing processes and the volatility and pathology of female reproductive processes (Schiebinger, 2013), the bodies of 'other women' (black, poor) were often regarded as brute matter—uncivilized, carnal and animal-like. The twin bifurcating process of 'naturalizing' African/indigenous women and 'civilizing' white women was a core feature of European colonization in which indigenous women became 'savages' and white women became 'ladies' (Mies, 2014).

In the present day, racist and imperialist prejudices about women's birthing bodies continue to underpin contemporary rhetoric about biomedicalization, 'natural childbirth' and rights-based discourse advocating for women's right to choice and control. These underlying assumptions are rarely recognized or acknowledged. Colonial ideas about indigenous and black women's bodies as primitive and animal-like and thus primed to give birth (and breastfeed) easily and without pain or the need for medical assistance, are rooted in ideologies of racial difference and Social Darwinism (Schiebinger, 2013). The first stories of primitive women giving birth without pain or difficulty date back to traveller's tales of the seventeenth and eighteenth century (Searle, 1965; Cosslett, 1994; Jasen, 1997). Similar beliefs were also held about poor women in broader Europe (Jasen, 1997). These conceptualizations of African, indigenous and black women's bodies have had destructive material effects and were used to justify poor quality of biomedical health care services for pregnant indigenous women in colonial contexts (Searle, 1965; Jasen, 1997). At the same time, traditional and indigenous approaches to birth (traditional birth attendants and midwives) were often denigrated, eroded and forcibly 'medicalized' through colonial impositions in many African contexts (Searle, 1965; Thomas, 2003). As a result, in many areas of the Global South, health care provision for pregnant and birthing women is uneven and often inadequate. Bifurcated obstetric systems, which offer different kinds of care for poor and rich women, persist in many Southern settings (e.g. South Africa, Brazil). Rates of avoidable maternal mortality continue to be unacceptably high in many areas of the Global South (particularly in sub-Saharan Africa) and global disparities in rates of maternal death stand as one of the most vivid and sobering examples of persistent inequality between countries of the Global South and North. Historical constructions of black birthing bodies as more 'primitive' and immune to pain have also been found to still resonate in the differential treatment of black/poor and white/privileged women's laboring bodies in the United States (see Bridges, 2011).

Colonial myths about easy and painless birth for so-called 'primitive' women also continue to frame and are used to legitimize the (largely middle-class and Euro-American) 'natural birth' movement and meta-narrative. The philosophy of birth articulated by British obstetrician Grantly Dick-Read in the 1930s and 1940s became a key text inaugurating the movement towards 'natural birth' from the 1950s and 1960s onwards. Dick-Read's natural birth philosophy was founded on racist distinctions between the bodily experience of birth for 'primitive' (i.e. black and poor) and 'civilized' (white and privileged) women. Difficulties, complications and pain during birth were seen as more prevalent among white, Euro-American women while black and poor women were regarded as uncontaminated by civilization and thus able to give birth unassisted and without pain (see Dick-Read, 1963). The tension/s between civilized minds and reproductive bodies (mind–body dualism) was regarded as a problem for white, middle-class, 'civilized' women during birth; these women thus needed to learn how to relax via the various techniques offered by 'natural childbirth' proponents (ironically also often male obstetricians) such as Dick-Read and Lamaze. Black and poor women were more 'bodily' and thus did not have the same tensions and conflicts between mind/body and were able to give birth easily and painlessly. These racist assumptions continue to resonate in contemporary discourse about homebirth, natural birth and unassisted birth or what has become known as 'free birth' in the form of the caricature of the 'Third World,' rural or 'primitive' woman who does not require biomedical assistance but gives birth alone and without medical intervention. According to Cosslett (1994, p. 9), the 'primitive' woman, "haunts western women's birth stories" as a romanticized, racist ideal that valorizes the power of the instinctive, pure or 'natural' birthing body that exists somewhere beyond or outside of sociocultural relations. This haunting can be seen in women's everyday stories about birth (Klassen, 2001) and in classic second-wave birth activist texts, which have in some cases become almost like bibles for the homebirth movement (see Arms, 1977). The trope of the primitive woman who approaches the birth of her baby in an 'uncomplicated' fashion, with a "built-in knowledge of childbirth" and "without fear" (Arms, 1977, p. 11) has been found to inspire and embolden women's decisions to birth outside the medical system (i.e. homebirth or unassisted birth) and pervade the talk of women planning homebirths (Klassen, 2001).

Although it is often assumed as such, the biological or 'natural' birthing body is not one thing or a universal phenomenon. Instead, constructions of the birthing body are entangled with racist ideas, discriminatory practices and colonial myths about the reproductive bodies of women from different class and race positions. These racialized ontological politics are enacted during birth, with the result that some birthing bodies are 'medicalized' and subject to many interventions and painkillers while others are framed as not needing pain relief or medical surveillance (see Chapter 4). Ontological politics matter, shaping the ways birth materializes in different settings. In the following section, I argue that essentialist and dualist understandings of the body that births are not just prevalent in biomedical and feminist interpretations, but that psychological research on birth is often founded on similar assumptions, thereby reinscribing dualisms and often unable to capture the psychofleshy complexities of birthing.

Psychological frames

Similarly to biomedicine, mainstream psychology continues to be embedded in a range of dualisms. The core object of psychological knowledge production has traditionally been 'the individual,' 'the mind' or personal sense of self and identity. Influenced by social constructionism, critical and feminist currents in psychology have challenged the individualism, binary thinking and decontextualized approach inherent in mainstream psychology over the last three to four decades (Henriques et al., 1998). Birth has not traditionally been a key topic of investigation in psychology (in feminist or mainstream psychology). In general, the work that has been done largely ignores feminist critiques of medicalization and is predominantly concerned with birth as a potential source of individual pathology or with the 'factors' associated with birth satisfaction, such as control and social support (see Weaver, 1998; Ayers & Pickering, 2005; Saxbe, 2017). While a robust corpus of feminist psychological work exists on other aspects of reproduction and childbearing (i.e. pregnancy and mothering), there has been an interesting lack of psychological engagement with *birth*.

In general, psychological research has tended to explore pre-birth (pregnancy) and post-birth (mothering) experiences, with birth often ignored. Many classic studies of the 'transition to motherhood' in psychology have thus treated birth as an incidental and insignificant event that only deserves a couple of superficial paragraphs (see Shereshefsky & Yarrow, 1973; Breen 1975; Leifer, 1977; Stern & Bruschweiler-Stern, 1998). Psychological literature has often approached pregnancy and motherhood as important 'feminine' developmental processes integral to the successful attainment of mature female identity (e.g. Chertok, 1969). Pregnancy and motherhood have thus been seen as developmental tasks that women either succeed or fail at. For some psychologists, birth has been construed as the dramatic 'peak' of the maternity 'crisis' (Chertok, 1969; Doering, Entwisle & Quinlan, 1980) in which psychic conflicts have to be resolved in order to be a 'good mother.' Women that fail to resolve these conflicts are seen as at risk for the perpetuation of damaging mother–infant relations (Doering, Entwisle & Quinlan, 1980; Durik et al., 2000). Conceptualizing motherhood as a series of developmental tasks necessary for successful 'adjustment' translates readily into the pathologization of pregnancy, birth and motherhood. Psychologists have tended to focus on pathology and dysfunction in relation to reproduction and motherhood, with substantial research focusing (for example) on postnatal depression and menstrual disorders. Feminist psychologists have critiqued the pathologization of women's reproductive experiences, with excellent work countering the pathologization of menstruation, maternity and the menopause (see Ussher, 1989, 2006; Nicolson, 1998, 1999; Hollway, 2015). Feminist psychologists have, however, for the most part avoided engaging with birth, with little critical feminist research conducted in this area (but see Baker, Choi & Henshaw, 2005; Ussher, 2006; Crossley, 2007; Shaw & Kitzinger, 2007). The tendency to assume that birth is an event of the biological body—all body and no mind—could underpin the lack of engagement by (feminist) psychologists. Limited conceptualizations of bodies as essentially biological entities, and thus outside the remit of psychological investigation, continue to pervade mainstream academic psychology. A psychology of birth thus might seem to many to be a contradiction in terms.

As a result, psychologists have had little to say about birth as a subjective, psychofleshy experience, preferring to focus on potential psychological disorders associated with birth. Psychological work has thus focused on birth as both a source of irrational and pathological fear and a possible site for the development of trauma and post-traumatic stress syndrome (PTSD). For example, tokophobia, defined as "an unreasoning dread of childbirth" (Hofberg & Brockington, 2000, p. 83) was classified as a psychological disorder in 2000 and is associated with a range of other psychological problems including anxiety, depression, PTSD and bonding disorders. There is a tendency for psychological research on both 'fear of childbirth' and birth-related PTSD to focus solely on individual risk factors, situated inside the woman, as the primary source of fear and trauma. For example, pain-avoiding behavior has been associated with a 'neurotic' personality, "unconscious aggressive feelings towards the child" or an unplanned pregnancy (Saisto & Halmesmäki, 2003, p. 203). Problems, fears and anxieties associated with birth are thus often decontextualized and divorced from sociomaterial and ideological issues.

Driven by the goal to improve maternity services, some researchers have been trying to isolate the 'factors' associated with birth satisfaction since the 1980s. The following factors have been linked to satisfaction with birth: social support (Doering, Entwisle & Quinlan, 1980; Fox & Worts, 1999; Waldenström et al., 2004), personal control and decision-making (Fowles, 1998; VandeVusse, 1999; Gibbons & Thomson, 2001; Green & Baston, 2003), discrepancies between expectations and reality (Gibbins & Thomson, 2001; Ayers & Pickering, 2005), pain (Fowles, 1998; Hodnett, 2002), place of birth (Janssen, Carty & Reime, 2006; Christiaens & Bracke, 2009) and the type and degree of medical intervention (Waldenström, 1999; Waldenström et al., 2004). Unfortunately, most studies on birth satisfaction have been conducted with relatively homogenous samples of Euro-American, white, middle-class women. Furthermore, while a lot of this research has been qualitative, women's own stories and accounts of birth have often been simplified and 'made-to-fit' pre-existing conceptual grids (i.e. expectations versus reality, control, decision-making). 'Birth satisfaction' is itself arguably an abstract and imposed concept that reduces a complex, embodied experience into artificial, separable and discrete 'factors.' This amounts to 'thingification'— namely the process of turning complex relations into 'things' (see Barad, 2007). The birthing subject assumed and reproduced in studies of 'birth satisfaction' has been, in general, a disembodied individual and there has been little consideration of birth as a complex embodied and sociomaterial experience.

While psychology has offered limited insights into the psychological, subjective and embodied experience of birth (from the mother's perspective), psychoanalytic writing on birth has been richer. This is not surprising given that theorizing the significance of the body, its agentic forcefulness in the form of drives and erogenous zones, and the psychic representations of fleshy embodiment, have always been important psychoanalytic concerns. While the psychic implications and significance of women's reproductive, pregnant and birthing bodies are often muted in psychoanalytic work (Balsam, 2012) and marginalized in Freudian theory, there has been some interesting writing by women psychoanalysts on the psychic complexities and implications of birth (e.g. Deutsch, 1944; Kristeva, 1986b). In particular, the writing of Joan Raphael-Leff (1991, 1993) has powerfully explored the ontological complexities and challenges that the fleshy act of giving birth poses for women. In contrast to most mainstream psychological work, the birthing body-subject that appears in her writing is a flesh and blood, pulsating, hurting, erotic and complex embodied self. Birth is acknowledged as "a deeply arousing experience" (p. 223) involving "pain, blood, mess, naked emotionality and urgency" (p. 224). The birthing woman is powerfully embodied, active and emotionally effusive in Raphael-Leff's writing and she notes "her suffering, her ecstatic reactions or excessive screaming, her whimpering, crying out, beseeching or groping." This is the 'loud body' that births (Shabot, 2016) often sanitized and silenced in birth scholarship and research. Raphael-Leff's (1991, 1993) work is rare in providing extensive engagement with the birthgiver's potentially paradoxical, intense, psychofleshy perspectives of pregnancy, labor and birth. The psychic meanings of the body that births, its relation to the primordial mother and the bodily challenges that birthing woman potentially have to negotiate (between separation and unity, letting go and holding on, splitting and cohesion) are bravely explored by Raphael-Leff (1991).

Silenced in most psychological research, the psychofleshy experiences of birthing have been well articulated by women writers (such as Anäis Nin, Phyllis Chesler, Margaret Atwood and Doris Lessing), poets (i.e. Sharon Olds, Audre Lorde and Toi Derricotte) and feminist philosophers (see Young, 1990a; Battersby, 1998; Lintott & Sander-Staudt, 2012; LaChancee Adams & Lundquist, 2013). In the work of these writers, the fleshy and fragmented psychophysical experience of labor/birth is foregrounded. Birth comes alive as a bodily emotional process involving complex relations between flesh, feelings, relations, spaces, things, imaginings and meanings. Alice Adams (1994) shows, in her Lacanian inspired analysis, that women writers represent birth as an ontological and subjective bodily crisis in which bodies are shattered and selves are profoundly challenged. Birth emerges as a psychofleshy event in which women "radically reorganize their subjectivity" (Adams, 1994, p. 25); it is a space of "inward divisions" (p. 27), "expanding consciousness" (p. 29) and "expanded identities" (p. 28) in which the birthing woman "multiplies identities" (p. 27). Unfortunately, in most psychological research on birth (even when based on women's stories and experiences), the ambivalences, contradictions, ontological complexities and embodied realities of giving birth are erased. This is a result of the persistence of meta-theoretical binaries framing research, limited theoretical conceptualizations of bodies (seen predominantly as biological, natural and/or biomedical) and inadequate methodological strategies.

Birth politics and global activisms

Birth is highly political and situated at the center of ideological and moral struggles about women's bodies, maternity, biopolitics and reproduction. It is thus not surprising that birth has been the subject of Euro-American activisms for more than a century (see Beckett, 2005). More recently, the global politics of birth activism has mushroomed, diversified and splintered into a number of factions that defy easy categorization (Vissing, 2017). The ideal of the 'natural' or 'normal' (physiologically driven and unmedicated) birth, however, still functions as a core ideal of many activist groups (particularly those headed by professional midwives). Global birth activism is made up of a number of diverse organizations, groups and movements in a range of cross-national contexts, including professional midwifery organizations and groups, proponents of unassisted birth, the 'orgasmic birth' movement, homebirth movement, legislative advocacy groups, human rights in birth (also known as the 'humanizing birth' movement), safe motherhood initiatives and activists advocating against 'obstetric violence.'

Despite the proliferation of birth activisms, there is little consensus about what shape birth politics should take or what activists should be advocating *for* in relation to birth. There are thus varied and contested beliefs about what matters most in relation to birth (i.e. outcomes, safety, the fulfillment of ideal femininity, ecstasy and spirituality, human rights, individual choice or the absence of 'medicalization') and how birth should 'ideally' unfold. At the core of these tensions are volatile ideological, political and conceptual contestations or 'ontological politics' about femininity, women's bodies, maternity and geopolitics. There are also substantial differences in the kinds of birth politics materializing in Northern and Southern settings. In the North (and in Southern contexts of privilege), birth debates often revolve around tensions between the valorization of individual choice, the idealization of unmedicated, 'normal' birth and the critique of medicalization. In these contexts, the idea of the 'perfect' birth is a powerful regulatory ideal (Rossiter, 2017; Vissing, 2017). According to this ideal, women *should* experience birth as empowering, pleasurable and exultant. In Southern contexts, birth politics and activisms often involve questions of human rights in birth, reproductive justice, safe birth and improvements in medical care, and issues of mistreatment and violence (including obstetric violence).

Idealizing 'normal birth'

As I will argue throughout this book, birth is ontologically contested with a number of competing concepts defining the parameters of what birth *is* or *should be*. The idea of 'normal birth' functions as one of these key ontological concepts and is invoked and valorized by many birth activists. While widely used by midwives and birth workers and often regarded as the alternative to interventionist birth, the parameters of 'normal' birth are in actuality defined by obstetric norms. The concepts of normality and abnormality in relation to birth have historically been defined by obstetrics, with the scope for 'normality' becoming ever narrower in the context of rising biomedical risk discourses (Scamell, 2011). While scholars have written cautionary pieces concerning the problems associated with terms such as 'normal birth' (see Darra, 2009; Lyerly, 2012), birth activists and midwives in

Northern settings continue to mobilize around this concept. For example, the International Normal Labor and Birth Conference has been an annual event since 2005 and midwives in the United Kingdom, Canada, New Zealand, America and Australia continue to actively promote 'normal birth' (see Darra, 2009). While good intentions underpin these endeavors, the use of terms such as 'normal birth' and 'natural birth' are deeply problematic (Lyerly, 2012). As argued by social theorists, the concept of 'normality' and 'the normal' are ideological and have often been mobilized in projects of oppression (see Foucault, 1979; Hacking, 1990).

Underpinning the idea of 'normal birth' is the assumption that the birthing body is primarily a physiological body that can be separated from sociomaterial relations, medical apparatus and practices. The term 'normal birth' also implies that unmedicated birth is the best, ideal or most desirable mode of birth and that technology is problematic and 'abnormal.' At the same time, the concept of 'normal birth' remains slippery. In obstetric practice, 'normal birth' is a retrospective category; all births are assumed abnormal until proven otherwise (Gould, 2000). Midwives commonly describe 'normal' birth as births characterized by "the *relative* absence of medical intervention" (Lyerly, 2012, p. 315; emphasis added). However, just how much and what kinds of medical interventions are 'allowed' for a birth still to be deemed 'normal' remains unclear. Some midwives have defined 'normal birth' as, "a purely physiological event with no interventions" (Gould, 2000, p. 419). However, the same midwives argue that the use of certain interventions such as the rupturing of membranes, induction and episiotomy would not necessarily make labor/birth abnormal (Gould, 2000). As argued in Chapter 3, even births that take place outside of the hospital system are often still framed in relation to normative biomedical scripts and expectations. There is thus no birth that is "a purely physiological event" (Gould, 2000, p. 419) standing apart from socio-cultural meta-narratives.

The dangers and exclusions of birthing idealizations

The idea of 'normal birth' is not just valorized by midwives but is also entangled with problematic and commodified idealizations of birth. In contexts of sociomaterial privilege, 'natural,' 'normal' and/or 'joyful' birth is often idealized, intersecting with neoliberal modes of consumption to make a 'pleasurable birth' into a commodity that women can achieve with the right preparation and paraphernalia (Rossiter, 2017). The idealization of 'normal birth' is also a problematic ingredient of some forms of Euro-American birth activism. According to Vissing (2017), the 'Birth Rights movement' has idealized unmedicated, non-interventionist modes of birth with problematic consequences for women. Birth has thus become reified in some circles as a revolutionary event that *should be* intrinsically positive and transformative or "wondrous, ecstatic and fulfilling" (Vissing, 2017, p. 174). Within such frames, medical assistance or technologies become barriers to the realization of 'authentic' birth. Some midwives and mothers are so opposed to any form of medical interference during birth that they promote ideals of 'unassisted' or 'free birth' as goal (Haydock, 2014) in which women are encouraged to give birth without midwives or medical attendants of any kind. Women are encouraged to "return to their natural selves" (Rossiter, 2017, p. 51) and eschew technocratic, cultural and biomedical 'distortions' of physiological birth. The idealization of 'normal' birth also intersects with moralistic messages about 'good' mothering and myths about an essential femininity based on an authentic bodily experience.

Underlying idealizing beliefs about 'authentic' birth as joyful, blissful and revolutionary are ontological assumptions about birthing bodies. Instead of being defective machines (i.e. biomedical view), birthing bodies become sources of transformatory bliss and 'authenticity.' Birthing bodies are assumed to be 'pure' physiologies apart from sociomaterial contexts, politics and relations. Birth is idealized as a benevolent experience (when done authentically) with unmedicated, 'physiological' birth constructed as a heady and blissful (potentially orgasmic) hormonal rush involving a 'feel good' combination of endorphins, oxytocin and prolactin. In order to realize their 'right' to a joyful birth, women need to trust 'the body' and trust the birthing process. While valorizing the birthing body as a positive source of empowerment, dualism continues to pervade these kinds of idealizations. According to Vissing (2017), such idealizations dispel anxiety about the uncertainties associated with the (birthing) body by constructing the physiological process of birth as inherently good, safe and benevolent. However, by casting birth as a process that *can* unfold apart from sociomaterial politics, these idealizations underestimate the power of risk discourses and overestimate women's capacities to 'empower' themselves as individual agents in the face of a powerful socioeconomic/biomedical/neoliberal machinery or 'medical industrial complex' (Rossiter, 2017). Idealizations of 'normal' birth also construct physiological birth as a universally 'good' and singular experience, disregarding the forceful fleshy corporeality of birthing, which can be painful, overwhelming and threatening.

On the other side of these idealizations also lie racial, classed and other *exclusions* based on various modes of social marginalization (i.e. sexuality, ableism). It is white mothering (within a heterosexual marriage) that has historically been regarded as 'good,' joyful and beneficial to society while black maternity and fertility have often been cast as deviant, suspicious and troublesome (Bridges, 2011). Black women have also historically been constructed as closer to nature (than white women), hyper-fertile, characterized by 'obstetrical hardiness' and 'primitive pelvises' (Hoberman, 2005) that enable them to give birth effortlessly and without the need for pain relief or medical intervention. These racist myths continue to shape beliefs about black pregnant and birthing bodies (Bridges, 2011). The call to return to 'authentic' birth and "natural selves" (Rossiter, 2017, p. 51) while ostensibly neutral, is actually an implicitly racially marked project aimed at predominantly white and privileged women. Idealizations of certain types of birth (i.e. unmedicated and 'joyful') also intra-act with neoliberal bioeconomics, so that the responsibility for achieving 'perfect birth' belongs to the birthing woman (and her partner). Idealizations of 'the perfect birth' silence issues that might prevent poor or marginalized women from satisfying and empowering births (i.e. structural inequalities, lack of basic resources, unsafe environments).

Human rights violations

Since the 2000s, a growing body of birth activism has focused on human rights and birth. An editorial by midwife Jan Tritten in 2009 argued that women's rights *as human beings* were often violated during birth. Rights to bodily autonomy, freedom of choice and humane, dignified treatment often seem to vanish during pregnancy, labor and birth, particularly in medicalized settings. Multiple onto-logical tensions underlie the easy disappearance of these human rights. First, there is an inherent tension between the concept of 'human rights' and pregnancy/birth because the prototypical 'human being' embedded in rights discourse is often based on a male prototype. Pregnancy, labor and birth defy masculinist concepts of the disembodied, singular human being who is separate and distinct from others. The birthgiver is not one but two. The multiplicity and indeterminacy of pregnant and birthing embodiment challenges individualist conceptions of human rights, particularly given that the interests of mother and infant are often regarded as competing and at odds in biomedical frameworks. Second, the role of the patient is embedded in a hierarchical authority relation whereby medical experts, doctors and nurses are seen as imbued with authoritative knowledge (Jordan, 1993). The patient identity thus arguably exists in tension with the notion of the free indi-vidual agent with 'rights.'

Despite these conceptual tensions, activists, academics and practitioners have applied the rhetoric of 'human rights' to fight for improvements in maternity care. Since 2010, an annual Birth Rights conference has been held and various global organizations (e.g. Global Midwifery Council, Human Rights in Childbirth, White Ribbon Alliance, International MotherBaby Childbirth Organization) have been founded which focus on treatment during birth as a human rights issue. Many have applied the FREDA principles (fairness, respect, equality, dignity and autonomy), ethical values used as part of a broader human rights approach to health care in the UK, as ethical ideals for maternity practice. From a global perspective, human rights in birth also include the right to safe motherhood and needed medi-cal care. According to Fathalla (2006, p. 409), the high rates of maternal deaths in the Global South are, "the ultimate tragic outcome of the cumulative denial of women's human rights."

The rhetoric of 'human rights' in birth is important but lacks sustained engage-ment with the implications of the fleshy corporeality of birth. The values and principles often espoused by a rights-based approach—i.e. autonomy, freedom of choice, dignity, fairness and respect are often articulated as free-floating, abstract and disembodied concepts. Problematically, the ontological frames shaping vocab-ularies of 'human rights' are implicitly molded on the prototype of the male, Cartesian subject—who has the right to 'self-determination' and the freedom to make choices and enact individualist autonomy apart from sociomaterialities and fleshy corporeality. Rights-based activisms need to build values and principles based on alternative ontologies that take corporeality seriously.

Humanizing birth and countering violations

The 'humanizing birth movement' has emerged as an international activist movement that is particularly strong in Latin American contexts (e.g. Brazil). 'Humanizing' birth means "considering women's values, beliefs, and feelings" (Behruzi et al., 2010) and treating birthgivers as human persons rather than machines (Wagner, 2001; Rattner, 2008). In 2001, Robbie Davis-Floyd outlined the 'humanistic' approach to birth as an alternative mode to the technocratic and holistic paradigms. According to Davis-Floyd (2001, p. 10), underpinning the humanistic model is a drive towards humanizing medicine—that is, an effort "to make it relational, partnership-oriented, individually responsive and compassionate." In relation to birth, the goal is to make maternity care "more loving" (p. 10) and humane and to foster caring and respectful relations between birthgivers and health care providers. While some work within the humanizing birth approach to humanize obstetrics while still endorsing technology and standard obstetric protocols (see Davis-Floyd, 2001), others regard medicalized birth as "necessarily dehumanizing" (Wagner, 2001, p. S26). According to Rattner (2008), the humanizing approach is critical of the mechanistic treatment of birth (i.e. treating the birthing body as machine or biomedical object) and focuses both on highlighting the psychological aspects of interpersonal relations between birthgivers and health care providers and the links between dehumanized and depersonalized maternity care and institutional violence. Importantly, Rattner (2008, p. 6) notes that the rhetoric of humanization is "a less accusatory and strategic term to talk with healthcare professionals about institutional violence."

Some Latin and Central American birth activists have however shifted from using the language of 'humanizing birth' to the far more overtly political terminology of 'obstetric violence' (Pérez D'Gregorio, 2010; Dixon, 2015; Pickles, 2015; Diaz-Tello, 2016). While violations during labor/birth are often framed with/in vocabularies of 'trauma' in Northern settings (see Mozingo et al., 2002; Moyzakitis, 2004; Baker, Choi & Henshaw, 2005; Thomson & Downe, 2008; Elmir et al., 2010), activists in Southern contexts are leading the way in naming mistreatment during birth as a form of violence against women—i.e. 'obstetric violence.' Importantly, both the 'humanizing birth' movement and activist work around 'obstetric violence' recognize that mechanistic models of birth (and birthing bodies) are implicated in interpersonal violations, dehumanized care and mistreatment during labor/birth. While the 'humanizing birth' movement focuses on a critique of normative biomedical models of birth, obstetric violence activists have embraced an intersectional approach in which biomedicine is seen as intertwined with race, class and gendered modes of marginalization. However, both movements are in danger of repudiating technology and obstetric interventions as inherently disempowering (see Wagner, 2001) and slipping back into unreflexive idealizations of 'normal' or 'natural' birth and valorizations of disembodied notions of 'autonomy' and 'choice' (see Pérez D'Gregorio, 2010).

Continuities in experiences of violation during labor/birth in maternity services across a range of geopolitical settings (see Beck, 2004; D'Ambruoso, Abbey & Hussein, 2005; El Nemer, Downe & Small, 2006; Elmir et al., 2010; Dzomeki, 2011; Ghani & Berggren, 2011; Mselle et al., 2011; Forssén, 2012) suggest that this is not just a problem of stressed systems, lack of evidence-based practices or medical technologies and interventions. Instead, violations are inextricably linked to broader sociomaterial disrespect for birthing bodies. This pervasive disrespect is not tied to technology or medical intervention per se, but is embedded in (historical and sociomaterial) biomedical onto-epistemologies and gendered, racialized and classed power relations. Ontological assumptions about birthing bodies and birthgivers— what they *are* (i.e. machines, disembodied objects, abject bodies, patients without rights) and what *matters most* in relation to birth (i.e. physical outcome, life/death, the reiteration of authoritative knowledge) shape relations in birth assemblages. Patriarchal prejudices and denigrating beliefs about women's bodies have been intertwined with biomedicine via a long historical process (Moscucci, 1990). Intersectional and geopolitical diffractions also impact on the ways in which particular women (poor, black, disabled, queer, transwomen) are treated, resulting in discontinuities in the ways in which violations manifest in different settings. Oppressive ontological beliefs about birth, women's reproductive and birthing bodies and the subjectivity and humanity of birth need to be tackled if oppressive relations and mistreatment during birth are to be addressed (see Chapter 7).

Northern feminist politics: disembodiment and 'choice'

Sociomaterial, geopolitical and intersectional differences in the ways in which birthing bodies are conceptualized, regulated and treated have been largely ignored in feminist research on birth (but see Dillaway & Brubaker, 2006; Brubaker, 2007; Johnson, 2016). The feminist politics of birth has traditionally been embedded in Northern perspectives and has foregrounded the experiences of middle-class, Euro-American women. While sharply critical of the biomedicalization of birth in the 1970s and 1980s, from the 1990s onwards, feminist rhetoric (centered in the geopolitical North) began to embrace and emphasize women's agency and 'choice' in relation to birth. While the feminist critique of medicalized birth has persisted (see Wolf, 2013), issues of agency, choice and the birthing woman as consumer have become important themes. In the 1990s, it was reported that some Euro-American women were comfortable and satisfied with obstetric technology and medicalized birth experiences (Fox & Worts, 1999; Davis-Floyd, 2003). These women were happy to be 'technocratic bodies' (Davis-Floyd, 1994) and welcomed the use of technology as a path to control and empowerment in birth. As a result, there were calls for sociologists of birth to move away from passive conceptualizations of birthing women as victims of medicalization and patriarchal medicine, and look at women's resistance and agency (Annandale & Clark, 1996;

Zadoroznyj, 1999). Birthing women in contexts of the Global North became positioned in birth scholarship as reflexive and autonomous agents or 'consumers' making choices about birth amidst an array of expert plural-knowledges. The pregnant body was no longer just a biomedical object but also a 'reflexive body' (Williams & Bendelow, 1998) or 'body-project' central to middle-class birth and mothering as identity-making and consumer projects (Taylor, 2000, 2008; Taylor, Layne & Wozniak, 2004). Birth and maternity care were reconceptualized in relation to a plethora of choices or "profusion of possibilities" in terms of both service providers and settings (Zadoroznyj, 1999, p. 268). The authority of biomedical knowledge was thus ostensibly decentered and attention shifted to women's own sense of choice and agency (Zadoroznyj, 1999; Root & Browner, 2001).

For some feminists, consumerism in birth is read as a challenge to medical dominance (i.e. Zadoroznyj, 2001), while others argue that the shift to conceptualizing women as consumers rather than patients is derivative of the intersections between biomedicine and neoliberal economic agendas (Fannin, 2003). Fannin (2003) thus questions the emergence of the rhetoric of birth consumerism and 'choice' in the context of rising (global) medical interventions in hospital birth settings. Furthermore, a discourse of consumer choice (exemplified by middle-class practices such as a written 'birth plan') does not necessarily result in autonomy or embodied agency in the hospital (Shaw, 2002; Fannin, 2003; Crossley, 2007; Malacrida & Boulton, 2014). Feminist psychologist Michele Crossley (2007) reflects on some of these issues in her autobiographical piece. She grapples with the question of whether women truly do have the ability to make personal 'choices' about birth, particularly in the institutional spaces in which most women give birth. Risk discourses, the authoritative knowledge of medical experts, machines and technology, and the sociomaterial geography of medical spaces (often set up for things to go wrong), are powerful agentic forces during birth. Despite being socioeconomically privileged and educated about feminist arguments and medicalized birth, Crossley (2007) concludes that in her case the ability to make 'choices' during birth was minimal. She remains ambivalent about the reasons for this lack of choice and unsure whether her emergency caesarean was life saving or unnecessary. She is also reluctant to put the blame on 'medicalized birth.' As she says, "I still do not know if I should be challenging medicalization or not" (p. 559). Instead of critiquing 'medicalization' as a set of sociomaterial and discursive practices that produce constrained selves, Crossley (2007) argues that the rhetoric of 'choice' should be qualified in relation to 'risks' and that women should not be led to believe that all births will unfold 'naturally' and without complications just because women 'choose' or desire it. In the end, Crossley (2007) describes her birth as a lesson in recognizing the 'situated immanence' (i.e. bodily nature) of birth and the illusion of rhetoric that assumes that birthing women can 'choose' a natural or uncomplicated birth. Valorizing 'choice' and the enactment of 'agency' during birth is based on the assumption that 'agency' is something that one 'has' or does not have and that is exercised by individual, decontextualized selves on the basis of rational, pre-existing and coherent preferences (Zadoroznyj, 1999).

Ebert (1996) reminds us that the valorization of the 'rational individual' or "bourgeois isolate" (p. 242) is necessary to the reproduction of hegemonic socioeconomic structures—what she terms 'capitalist patriarchy' and what others would now refer to as neoliberal economic agendas. Obstetrics is not situated outside of these socioeconomic forces and has been instrumental in transforming the middle-class birthing women from a patient into a 'consumer' (see Fannin, 2003). Fannin (2003) provides an analysis of the emergence of 'home-like' birthing suites in American hospitals, showing how the development of alternative birthing spaces is inseparable from neoliberal economics. Shifting economic landscapes "are intimately bound to interpellations of new subjectivities around birth" (p. 515). The popularization of choice rhetoric and the assumption that women are now active consumers (rather than passive patients) is based on a number of problematic conceptualizations and erasures. First, as already alluded to, the rhetoric of 'choice' is based on a decontextualized and disembodied conception of the birthing woman as an individual agent who exercises rational choices divorced from social, political, economic and bodily contexts. This is the transcendent self (forged in mind–body dualism) who is 'in control' of their body. The body is mute, materializing predominantly as an object or project to be used and fashioned in identity work. Feminists have historically struggled for, and celebrated, women's right to make autonomous choices about their bodies. As a result, reclaiming the body or 'taking our bodies back' has long been a rallying call for feminist activism. The right to autonomy in relation to bodies stands as one of the core tenets of modern feminism (see Diamond, 1994). However, underlying the move to ground freedom in control over the body lies a problematic belief in the power of 'instrumental rationality'— that is: the belief that the rational mind can conquer both the body and nature (Diamond, 1994). Mind–body dualism thus often underpins the rhetoric of 'choice.'

The valorization of individual 'choice' and agency in relation to birth, while masquerading as a universal ideal, is also rooted in the perspectives of middle-class, white, and Euro-American women. Reducing the feminist politics of birth to questions of choice works to depoliticize feminist critique (Beckett, 2005) and narrowly ignores issues that concern women from contexts of the Global South. As argued by Segal (1994), the language of 'choice' "inevitably downplays social constraint and inequality" and usually "serves conservative ends more readily than progressive ones" (p. 305). It amounts to white, middle-class feminism once again unreflexively speaking for all women and dismissing the problems facing women in other contexts in which global legacies of inequality and colonization have resulted in persistently high rates of maternal mortality, uneven medicalization and often inhumane treatment during birth. Instead of speaking to these issues and trying to articulate a feminist politics of birth that is able to think through transnational and intersectional birth politics, many Western feminists continue to act as though all women are neoliberal subjects in privileged contexts able to exercise 'choices' and 'agency.' Instead of being universal desires, the ability to exercise 'choice,' 'agency' and 'control' in relation to birth have in fact been found to be predominantly concerns of middle-class women (see Johnson, 2016). Working-class women have been found to be more concerned about the availability of basic and continuous maternity care than exercising 'choice' or 'control' (Nelson, 1983).

Feminist researchers in the Global North have critiqued a biomedical view of birthing bodies, but have struggled to resist dualist modes of thinking about birthing bodies. As a result of difficulties in finding alternative (non-dualist) ways of conceptualizing birthing bodies and subjectivities, the Nothern feminist politics of birth has become limited in the twenty-first century. While activist efforts to demedicalize birth were extremely successful in the Global North from the 1960s to 1980s, resulting in birth reforms, the elimination of certain non-evidence based practices (i.e. routine perineal shaving and enemas) and more options for birthing women, feminist politics has been constrained by the continued dominance of middle-class and Euro-American perspectives. Powerful birth activist movements are currently at work in Latin and Central American contexts. Unfortunately, the work of Southern and Northern feminists and activists often seem to operate as separate silos in relation to birth politics, with different agendas, rhetoric and terminology. There is much scope for the development of transnational forms of birth activism across these divides. Currently, however, the feminist politics of birth in the Global North seems to have increasingly slipped into a problematic rhetoric of 'choice' (Beckett, 2005). As argued, this rhetoric intersects with neoliberal economic agendas, the increasing hegemony of biomedical risk discourse and 'surveillance medicine' (see Armstrong, 1995), as well as the erasure of issues facing women who are not situated in privileged positionalities.

Narrow and problematic assumptions about the ontologies of birthing bodies thus continue to underpin research and activism in relation to birth (in Northern and Southern settings). These assumptions shape politics, practices and rhetoric. Failure to grapple with the meanings, complexities and implications of birthing corporeality has, to a large extent, characterized both feminist and social science research and birth activisms. Many have assumed that the birthing body is a biological body and either attempted to redefine this ('natural') body in empowering terms or upheld mind–body dualism by conceptualizing the birthing body as a reflexive project worked on by the rational, choosing self. Others have emphasized the cultural aspects of birth and largely avoided questions surrounding the ontology of birthing bodies. Few scholars have applied alternative frames to think about the complex corporeality of birthing bodies and the implications of this for activisms and birth politics. In the following section, I explore the work of feminist social science researchers who *have* grappled with the meanings of birthing bodies and attempted to think about birth in non-dualist terms.

Through Foucauldian frames: inscribing birthing bodies

Largely from the 2000s, a small number of researchers began to focus on the intersections between power and birthing bodies using Foucauldian theory. These researchers have been interested in the ways normative power relations (and discourses) are *inscribed* upon bodies that birth to construct 'disciplined' or 'docile' bodies. Embedded in constructionism, these studies reject the assumption that bodies are biological entities separate from relations of power and sociodiscursive meanings. Instead, bodies are seen as coming to matter (or not) in relation to sociocultural frames, discourses and ideologies. Feminist studies operating within a Foucauldian approach to bodies, power and birth have moved beyond earlier conceptualizations of power (i.e. biomedicine) as an oppressive force and are interested in exploring how birthing bodies actively materialize as products of sociocultural discourses. Biomedicine and gender are the two central forms of power explored in these studies. In their efforts to trace the *productive* aspects of biomedical power, researchers operating within Foucauldian approaches move outside of tendencies to either cast women as passive victims of biomedicine or neoliberal subjects exercising rational 'choices.'

Biomedical power reconceptualized

Instead of being purely oppressive, Foucauldian researchers have conceptualized biomedical power as operating through the micro-techniques of surveillance, monitoring and normalizing techniques rather than simply overt force (Arney, 1982). According to Arney (1982), obstetric biomedicine is not a monolithic and unchanging system but a shifting collection of discursive and material practices that have changed over historical time. Arney (1982) argues that the contemporary era of obstetrics constitutes a 'monitoring' period in which obstetric power is widely dispersed and there is no clear agent of control/domination. Medical power has thus shifted from oppressive top-down control to the all-seeing, "normalizing gaze" (p. 88) of panopticism. In this vein, Wendy Simonds (2002) explores obstetric time as a mode of discipline that interpellates birthing bodies. Plotted against the obstetric timetable and subject to constant monitoring, birthing bodies are disciplined and regulated via normalization and rendered either normal or abnormal. Deviations and dysfunctions are produced via arbitrary obstetric norms and timetables and a lexicon of risk renders interventions morally necessary. There is thus no need to 'force' interventions on women. According to Simonds (2002), obstetric power has not lessened in recent times; it has simply changed in style and tactics. According to these researchers, obstetric monitoring and surveillance are the new currents of obstetrical power (Arney, 1982; Simonds, 2002; Davis & Walker, 2013). Simonds (2002, p. 567) argues that contemporary forms of medical power are paradoxical and, "as medical supervision becomes increasingly omnipresent, it becomes less visible." Drawing on Foucault's use of the panopticon metaphor, Davis and Walker (2013) refer to the 'obstetric panopticon' as a mode of constant potential surveillance that ultimately produces pregnant and birthing women as self-policing subjects. Biomedical power has also been framed as a set of spatial configurations that work upon laboring and birthing bodies in hospital settings (Sharpe 1999; Davis & Walker, 2010b). The organization of space is regarded as infused with discursive meaning and active in shaping both birth practices and subjectivities. Obstetric space is filled with medical equipment, surgical supplies and alarm buttons, steel trolleys laden with instruments and dominated by the obstetric bed. Such spatial arrangements constrain women's bodily movements and behaviors and communicate messages that birth is a medical and risky event and that the birthing body is vulnerable and prone to break down without there being any need for an individual agent of control or domination (Davis & Walker 2010b). Birth scholars working within Foucauldian theory have thus been interested in forms of biomedical power and coercion that operate transindividually—through material practices, spatial arrangements, discursive inscription/s and normative timetables. Some researchers have asked interesting questions about the possible ways in which relations of biomedical power might impact on the physiological, bodily birth experience (see Maher, 2003) but there has been little concrete research exploring such interconnections.

While Foucauldian birth research has usefully reconceptualized biomedical power as productive and as operating via surveillance and self-regulation, most studies emerge from Northern contexts and are based on the experiences of privileged, Euro-American women. As a result, we do not know a great deal about how biomedical power and risk discourses materialize in different geopolitical spaces or how they intersect with other modes of sociomateriality (e.g. race). Writing from the South African context, Kruger and Schoombie (2010) suggest that obstetric power does not operate via panoptic surveillance and the all-seeing gaze in public sector maternity settings catering for poor, and predominantly black, patients. Here the medical gaze is often absent, patients get lost in corridors (see Gibson, 2004) and become invisible. Biomedical power is thus not separate from other modes of power (i.e. coloniality, race, gender). This is a point that has often been missed in existing Foucauldian birth scholarship. Furthermore, more work needs to explore the logics of both visibility and *invisibility* in relation to operations of (biomedical) power (see Chapter 4). While articulations of race and coloniality vis-à-vis biomedical birth have not been widely explored in Foucauldian inspired research, researchers have explored *gender* as a form of disciplinary power that intersects with biomedicine.

Gendered bodies, femininities and birth

A small number of researchers have moved beyond an analytic focus on biomedicine as the primary form of power in relation to birth and have explored gender as a mode of bodily discipline (see Martin, 2003; Carter, 2009; Malacrida & Boulton, 2012; Chadwick & Foster, 2013; Shabot, 2016). They have argued that birth is not an isolated, decontextualized event that is only subject to forms of medicalized power. Rather, birth is a sociocultural event in which multiple forms of power coalesce. Researchers have argued that birth is saturated with gender imperatives and meanings about femininity and the female body. Furthermore, birth is a critical interpellative space for the performance and 'doing' of gender and femininity. For example, Martin (2003) found that 'internalized technologies' of femininity disciplined women's bodies during birth. Women thus described "doing normative gender while birthing" (p. 61) trying to be polite, 'nice,' selfless and sensitive towards the needs of others while they were in labor. Privileging a selfless and relational mode of gendered subjectivity also resulted in women looking to their male partners "to describe, define and decide about their experiences during labor, even their bodily ones" (Martin, 2003, p. 63). Martin's (2003) study pointed to the importance of gendered modes of regulation and bodily inscription during the labor and birth process.

Constructionist and Foucauldian researchers have argued that women do not stop being socially interpellated selves during labor/birth and that birth is not outside of sociocultural relations of gendering. Women's birth experiences materialize in relation to 'internalized technologies' of gender and normative femininity. Carter (2009) found that embodied gender performances were complex during labor. Many of the American women in her sample made a point of engaging in traditional feminine activities during labor such as cooking and cleaning and were adamant that appropriately 'presentable' feminine bodies were maintained by shaving their legs and putting on make-up. Furthermore, the internalization of a outsider patriarchal gaze whereby, "woman lives her body as seen by another, by an anonymous patriarchal Other" (Bartky, 1990, p. 72), emerged in the work of both Martin (2003) and Chadwick & Foster (2013) as a key 'technology of gender' operating in middle-class (predominantly white) women's birth narratives. Martin found that women 'adopted the other's gaze' in narrating their birth experiences. As a result, most of the women defined the 'real' birth as that which was 'seen' from the outside. Several women therefore said that they felt like they had missed the 'real' birth because they were unable to 'see' what was happening. The external spectacle of birth, as viewed from the perspective of the onlooker or observer was thus privileged over the psychofleshy, tactile, feeling and sensing corporeality of birthing. This suggests that biomedical power relations are not the only forces of discipline operating on birthing women; as argued by Martin (2003, p. 60), "internalized technologies of gender regulate and discipline women as well."

While Martin (2003) found that 'technologies of gender' framed women's retrospective talk about their births, Chadwick and Foster (2013) found that a 'patriarchal optics' and phallocentric representations of childbirth shaped the choices middle-class pregnant South African women made in relation to birth. Similarly, Malacrida and Boulton (2012) found that Canadian women constructed choices about birth in relation to idealized modes of femininity and the feminine body. Childless women in particular viewed 'messy' vaginal birth as a threat to ideals of feminine embodiment as contained, clean and demure as well as a challenge to heteronormative 'sexiness.' Women were also interpellated by gender normative discourses of maternal selflessness. Paradoxical discourses of embodied femininity (e.g. sexy available bodies versus selfless maternity) were thus found to discipline women's idealized and real birth choices. Complex and contradictory sociocultural and moralistic meanings about women's bodies, birth and (middle-class) femininity have thus been found to shape birth choices as well as women's expectations and anticipatory feelings about birth.

The liminal, ambiguous and undecidable characteristics of birthing, in which normative assumptions about singular selves and bodily self-containment implode, make birthing bodies potentially abject and monstrous within masculinist social imaginaries. According to Oliver (1993, p. 57), birth is the "prototypical abject experience" in which identity is fundamentally troubled. It is an undecidable moment between subject and object, one and two, internal and external; it is "the unruly border, birth" (p. 57). Studies exploring the gendering of birth have found that representations of birth as involving abject and frightening modes of embodiment are not just to be found outside in masculinist and medicalized cultures but have been internalized by many women and function as 'internalized technologies' of gender that shape, constrain and produce birth choices and experiences. Shabot (2016, p. 231) argues that noisy and 'unruly' laboring/birthing bodies are, "antithetical to the myth of femininity," according to which appropriately feminine bodies should be contained, modest and orderly. While researchers have found that technologies of femininity often function as self-policing modes of discipline during birth, Shabot (2016) argues that they also function as external modes of discipline. For Shabot (2016), the mistreatment and violation of women during medicalized birth (see Chapters 5 and 7) works as a form of 'gender discipline' that punishes women for displaying unruly and disruptive forms of embodiment. The ideal medical body is passive, inert and mute (see Leder, 1992) and the potentially powerful and 'noisy' forms of embodiment evoked by the labor/birth process challenge and confront medicalized assumptions about good patient bodies (Chadwick, 2017b). Birthing bodies thus potentially trouble both ideal forms of normative feminine embodiment and medical object bodies. This once again suggests that forms of power are entangled in relation to birth and that biomedical, gender and other forms of sociocultural power relations need to be explored in relation to one another rather than as separate silos of power.

While explorations of the entanglements between birthing bodies and discursive and sociomaterial forms of power remain critically important, the studies explored above focus predominantly on bodies as disciplined and regulated by normative discourses and do not generally offer complex portraits of the lived, fleshy corporeality of birthing. We need research that is able to think bodies as simultaneously interpellated and constrained in/by particular sociomaterial assemblages *and* as fleshy capacities that affect, feel, ache, respond and resist. In the following section, I explore the small number of studies that have explored the fleshy ontologies of birthing via women's birth stories.

Telling fleshy ontologies of birth

While there has been a burgeoning theoretical and philosophical interest in women's fleshy and corporeal experiences of reproductive embodiment since the 1990s, few researchers have explored birth as a psychofleshy experience. Building on the work of Iris Marion Young (1990a) on pregnant embodiment, there has been a spate of qualitative studies exploring women's embodied experiences of pregnancy

(Lupton, 1999b; Schmied & Lupton, 2001a; Wynn, 2002; Earle, 2003; Warren & Brewis, 2004; Longhurst, 2005; Tyler, 2011; Nash, 2012) and breastfeeding (Blum, 1999; Stearns, 1999; Schmied & Lupton, 2001b; Bartlett, 2002; Hausman, 2007; Boyer, 2012). Given this widespread feminist interest in procreative bodies, it is surprising that few studies have focused on birth as an embodied, fleshy experience.

Splitting, fragmenting and multiplying: the psychofleshy birth experience

While constituting a small body of work, the qualitative studies (see Sbisà, 1996; Akrich & Pasveer, 2004; Chadwick, 2009, 2012; Carter, 2010; Lupton & Schmied, 2013) that have focused on the embodied aspects of women's birth experiences have delivered rich and insightful analyses. These studies have found that women narrate the corporeal experience of birth as a complex fleshy ontology involving distinctive forms of being and relating. Themes of fragmentation, multiple body–self relations and paradoxical forms of embodied subjectivity have surfaced as key elements in women's birth stories. These studies show that the bodies and selves reproduced in women's birth narratives are not univocal, singular or coherent. Instead, women's birth stories slip and slide between multiple modes of self and embodiment.

For example, in Akrich and Pasveer's (2004) analysis of over 70 European birth narratives, the embodied birth experience emerged in women's tellings as fragmented and multi-layered. The study found that there was no one type of birthing body or body–self relationship enacted during birth. Instead, the researchers found a complex plurality of birthing bodies produced in women's birth narratives. Three bodies emerged as central in women's stories, namely: the 'body-in-labor,' 'embodied self' and the 'body-without-boundaries.' In most stories, the two central actors during birth were the 'body-in-labor' and the 'embodied self.' According to Akrich and Pasveer, the 'body-in-labor' is the paining, all-consuming fleshy corporeality of birth experienced during labor spasms and contractions. While in everyday life, 'the body' often recedes into the background, in active labor it becomes a 'dys-appearing body' (Leder, 1990) that is powerfully present and potentially overwhelming—manifesting as the unavoidable and all consuming 'body-in-labor.' During labor, women had to find ways or strategies for dealing with this paining, overwhelming mode of embodiment (see also Sbisà, 1996). In Akrich and Pasveer's analysis, the 'embodied self' and 'body-in-labor' were described as a shifting and fluid relation in which women slid between being unified with their body (between contractions) to being in a state of fragmentation or dissociation in which the paining and contracting 'body-in-labor' threatened to overwhelm the embodied self. Using a different terminology, Carter (2010) found similar themes in her analysis of the body–self relations constructed in the birth narratives of middle-class American women. Three key bodies are identified in her study, namely: autonomous bodies, accommodating bodies and collaborating bodies. The autonomous body—similarly to the 'body-in-labor'—was the active and independent laboring body that seemed to act/perform independently and separately from the embodied self. Accommodating and collaborating bodies referred to modes of body–self relationality in which birthing women achieved some kind of harmony, unity, collaboration between body/self and a sense of embodied agency.

Birth has emerged as a fleshy event that potentially presents bodily and ontological challenges to selfhood and normative ways of being. According to Lupton and Schmied (2013) who explored representations of the birthing body and the infant's body in Australian women's birth narratives, the moment of birth is a potential challenge to individualist ideals of bodily containment and selfhood. Lupton and Schmied (2013) deftly trace the ontological dimensions of birthgiving via women's descriptions of shifting bodily and emotional modes of being during birth. The potential ontological insecurity and vulnerability associated with birth is revealed in this study as women describe fears of bodily disintegration and loss of boundaries as their bodies increasingly 'open' to the world. The relationship between the birthing woman and the 'body-being-born' was narrated by women as a complex, fleshy and fluid negotiation in which women grappled with the ambiguous complexities of inside-outside and self-other boundaries as the 'body-being-born' slipped in and out of their bodies. This process was articulated by women as emotionally challenging and potentially confronting as they tried to deal with the "conceptual strangeness" (p. 6) of birthing.

Collectively, these studies suggest that labor/birth is a complex psychofleshy event in which women have to negotiate multiple bodies and body–self relations. The fleshy body emerges as a powerful force during labor/birth and challenges everyday enactments of self in which bodies are take-for-granted and selves are masterful. The ways in which women negotiate these challenges and the potential for labor/birth to "radically reorganize . . . subjectivity" (Adams, 1994, p. 25) has begun to be explored via qualitative research. At the same time, more work is needed which explores birthing bodies as transversal psychofleshy enactments which are also embedded in a range of discursive, structural and sociomaterial relations. More complex theorizations of the entanglements between flesh, language and materiality are needed to ground this kind of work. We need to move beyond research that explores birthing bodies as *either* docile and disciplined *or* as lived fleshy experience (see Crossley, 1996).

Summary

This chapter has explored conceptualizations of birthing bodies in biomedicine, social science research, feminist politics and global birth activisms. While few studies have engaged with the corporeality of birth, ontological assumptions about what birthing bodies 'are' or 'should be' and how best to manage and treat them, pervade scholarship, activism, everyday birth practices and transnational debates. I argued that dualist understandings continue to plague thinking, research and activism in relation to birth. As a result, birth politics often center on problematic idealizations and valorizations of birthing bodies or are in danger of becoming depoliticized in/through the rhetoric of individual 'choice.' Failure to engage with the meanings, complexities and implications of birthing embodiment has been a consistent theme in research, debates and activism. Furthermore, there have been few attempts to use alternative frames to think through the corporeality of birth.

While dualist assumptions about birth pervade scholarship and politics, the few studies that have explored birthing corporeality have shown that birth is a complex psychofleshy experience involving multiple bodies and relations. These studies trouble assumptions that birthing bodies are simply biological entities separate from selves. According to Akrich and Pasveer (2004, p. 68), birth is a paradoxical dance or "pendulum movement" between the body-in-labor and the embodied self, with various body–self relations possible, depending on sociomaterial factors and the kind of medicalization involved. In some studies, the type and degree of medicalization was found to impact on the relationship between the 'body-in-labor' and the 'embodied self' (Akrich & Pasveer, 2004; Carter, 2010). Lupton and Schmied (2013) argue that the kind of birth a woman has (i.e. high degree of intervention, unmedicated or caesarean birth) is pivotal to how they experience the bodily emotional experience of birth. Importantly, findings suggest that there is not necessarily one (deleterious) meaning of medical intervention (see also Lyerly, 2006). For example, Akrich & Pasveer (2004) found that when intervention helped to facilitate an articulation or relation between the 'body-in-labor' and the 'embodied self' (for example, when internal sensations and external interpretations or measurements matched), medical intervention could be experienced as positive, affirming and empowering. At other times, women described medical interventions as producing a disempowering and damaging objectification of the 'body-in-labor.'

A common theme of women's narratives is that birth is often an event of duality or fragmentation and that women need to be embedded in supportive and affirming relational contexts in order to negotiate the psychofleshy challenges of birthing. Studies on birthing corporeality thus suggest that embodied relations are pivotal to women's feelings about their births. Akrich and Pasveer (2004) argue that it is the obliteration of the 'twosome' or duality of 'body-in-labor' and 'embodied self' that can result in a sense of alienation and disempowerment in relation to birth. Such obliterations can occur during certain types of birth (i.e. during surgical birth or birth with epidural) or emerge as the effects of unsupportive and violating birth assemblages (see Chapter 5). According to these studies, birth is an ontologically challenging psychofleshy experience that involves complex "internal negotiations" (Adams, 1994, p. 15) of splitting, pain, fragmentation and the loss of bodily boundaries. This underlines the importance of attending to the complexity of birthing corporeality in efforts to understand and improve women's birth experiences. The analytic chapters that follow explore the multiple enactments of birthing bodies within particular sociomaterial assemblages and aim to show both the lived corporeality of labor/birth and its entanglements in normative discourses, power relations, sociomaterial and relational assemblages.

3

CLOCKWORK BODIES

The focus of this chapter is biomedical ontologies of power and the ways they materialize as narrative scripts in women's birth stories. I am interested in the kinds of birthing bodies generated by these scripts/frames. I argue that biomedical power is not an external, generalized or totalizing force, but a set of everyday intra-acting relations (Barad, 2007) and ontological frames, materializing as particular narratives of birth and working on/through birthing bodies. While biomedicalization has often been understood as an oppressive or 'top-down' mode of power (Rothman, 1982; Martin, 1987; Michaelson, 1988), this chapter adopts a Foucauldian understanding of power as a force that "traverses and produces things, it induces pleasure, forms knowledge, produces discourse" (Foucault, 1984, p. 61). In line with new materialism, I argue further that biomedical power also produces ontologies of birth, materializing and shaping birthing bodies in particular forms. The chapter is interested in exploring the productive aspects of biomedical power as enacted in birth narratives. How does biomedical power produce particular ontologies of birth and birthing bodies? How is medical power potentially entangled with/in stories, bodies and experiences? How might biomedical power work differently on the bodies/narratives of women from different race and class positions?

This chapter proceeds by exploring the entanglements between performing and constructing birth narratives, and biomedical vocabularies and ontological frames. Birth narratives are not seen as pure reflections of experience or 'what really happened' but as diffracted in/though broader sociomaterial and biomedical frames. Biomedical power is both performatively produced, reiterated and subverted by women's birth narratives and simultaneously shapes and enables what can be said and narrated. Narrative and discourse are thus not simply what is said or told but, "that which constrains and enables what can be said" (Barad, 2007, p. 146). Furthermore, they also shape the kinds of birthing bodies produced in both event and research assemblages. Biomedical power is not simply an external authoritative force that acts in a uniform or top-down manner. Instead, it operates within birth assemblages intra-actively to enable modes of paradoxical agency, ways of knowing and produces desires. While biomedical modes of power can and do restrict, oppress and mute women's agency in some birth assemblages, biomedicalization also potentially enables forms of 'ambiguous agency' in relation to birth (Geerts & Van der Tuin, 2013). Biomedical power is, however, also always thoroughly intersectional, materializing in emergent 'birth assemblages' in which local norms, historical legacies and cultural storylines about race, class, age and gender intra-act with biomedical modes of discipline, surveillance, invisibilization and inscription. Focusing on women's stories shows that biomedical power does not just reside 'out there' as a mode of domination that is applied from the outside but that, in birth assemblages, it is also an emergent, intersectional, ontological and relational form of power produced by, and entangled with, local norms, cultural narratives, modes of technology, material institutions, patterns of sociocultural oppression and the fleshy materiality of birthing bodies.

In my analytic work, I found that biomedical ontologies dominated women's storytelling about birth. Biomedical frames became narrative and performative scripts that framed women's birth experiences and stories. I have called this biomedical narrative, as it materialized in women's stories, 'clockwork birth.' Clockwork narratives, defined as normative and medically derived storylines of birth, infiltrated and often colonized women's storytelling, producing particular ontologies of birth and birthing bodies and paradoxical forms of agency. The particular shape/configuration of clockwork narratives, however, differed according to sociomaterial positioning and mode of birth (i.e. different birth assemblages).

Clockwork birth

It was like clockwork, literally.

(Stephanie, white, planned homebirth)

Biomedical ontologies of birth served as dominant frames for telling birth stories. Having a story to tell about birth was, in most instances, heavily dependent on biomedical frames and interpretive devices. As a result, what I have called the 'clockwork narrative' was prominent in most women's efforts to make sense of birth. What exactly is a clockwork narrative of birth? The clockwork story is a cultural narrative derived from biomedical framings of labor/birth that provides an 'ideal' and formulaic script and plotline for the birth drama. It is thoroughly embedded in the ontological logic of biomedical norms and measurements in which birth is a measurable and linear physiological process. In the clockwork frame, birth is 'made sense of' by being plotted as a series of measurements in centimeters (degree of dilation), minutes (time lapse between contractions) and hours. Deeply ingrained in biomedical ontologies of birth, this narrative script is often reproduced in snippets on popular television shows and films; we all probably recognize the stereotypical image of the birthing couple who react to the possibility of labor by immediately hauling out the stop-watch and timing contractions. According to this obstetric script, 'normal' labor proceeds in a linear series of phases and follows a predictable and measurable trajectory. The clockwork script is to be found in birth preparation books and teachings at antenatal classes as well as women's writing about birth (i.e. Chesler, 1979). Birth, in this ontological frame, materializes as a linear process that can be measured and carved up in relation to obstetric timetables and norms.

Clockwork birth is thus based upon an ideal, 'textbook' medical version of 'normal birth,' which meets all the demands of biomedical norms; that is: the birth is not 'overdue,' the amniotic fluid breaks appropriately, labor contractions proceed in a regular, predictable and efficient manner (discerned by timing them) leading to the uncomplicated dilation of the cervix to ten centimeters (within an acceptable time-frame). Once full dilation is reached, the 'urge to push' is present and overwhelming and the baby is delivered spontaneously. Of course, this ideal textbook version of birth rarely materializes in medicalized settings, resulting in the 'need' for interventions and medical technologies. It is against the normative (and usually unattainable) ideal of clockwork birth that the birth process (and birthing bodies) are routinely measured, judged and deemed 'normal' or 'abnormal.' More often than not (particularly in hospital settings), clockwork birth goes awry and the birthing body 'malfunctions,' thereby necessitating medical interventions and confirming the patriarchal view that women's bodies are prone to 'break-down' and inherently dysfunctional (see Martin, 1987; Davis-Floyd, 2003). The normative clockwork script is based on Friedman's curve, a "time-motion statistical analysis" (Simonds, 2002, p. 565) of the different stages of labor, developed in the 1950s. Friedman's curve created a set of (arbitrary) norms whereby the progression of labor could be measured and 'deviations' identified and medically managed.

Clockwork birth, the normative medical textbook version of 'normal' birth, functioned as an ontological framing device or internalized technology of power that materialized particular kinds of birthing bodies and shaped birth narratives in powerful ways. Clockwork birth was also strongly *desired* by many of the women interviewed and many worked hard to try and fit their birth experience into this narrative and ontological frame. Surprisingly, even women choosing to birth at home were found to be strongly attached to making sense of their birth stories in relation to this biomedical ontology. The degree to which women were able to position themselves within a clockwork script and decode the birth experience via this framework was, however, not the same for all of the participants and differed substantially according to particular sociomaterial birth assemblages. While the clockwork narrative functioned as a mode of biomedical discipline, it also enabled middle-class homebirthers to enact forms of agency and control in relation to the birth experience. These women were given more access to biomedical modes of information from their health care providers (i.e. private midwives) about the progress of labor, degrees of dilation and potential complications, which they used to construct forms of embodied agency. Poorer women were often denied access to biomedical information from their health care providers and as a result, were often left unable to construct forms of agency in relation to the bodily experience of birth. The physiology and materiality of the labor/birth process itself, which unfolded in different and idiosyncratic ways, also affected the degree to which women were able to frame their experience within the ontological parameters of the clockwork narrative.

In the analysis that follows, I show how the clockwork narrative functioned as an internalized biomedical form of discipline entangled in birth stories and events, arguing that it also served intra-actively to shape, enact and materialize birth and certain kinds of birthing bodies. The birth event itself was often negotiated in relation to the frames and scripts offered by a broader clockwork narrative (diffracted by race/class). The fleshy and material experience of birth thus did not occur as a discrete physiological event separate from sociomaterial relations but was always already framed and constituted through ontological frames and plot-lines and societal relations of power. At times, however, depending on emergent relations, the fleshy materiality of birthing bodies spoke back and shattered the linear framework of the clockwork narrative. The biomedically derived clockwork script was internalized by many women as the normative ideal and was often intertwined with expectations of labor/birth. Problematically, the clockwork narrative is rooted in a biomedical ontology of birth and valorizes ways of knowing situated outside the birthing woman—i.e. the clock, dilation measurements and/or the medical expert.

Clockwork scripts and the muting of birthing bodies

How did clockwork birth, as a biomedical script for 'normal' birth, materialize in women's birth stories? Obviously, the specifics of the clockwork narrative intra-acted with mode of birth and the particularities of sociomaterial/relational birth assemblages. Ironically, the clockwork ideal was often most powerfully realized in (planned and privileged) homebirth assemblages, situated outside of the dominant machinery of medical technologies, experts and norms. Birth thus materialized as textbook, uncomplicated and 'like clockwork' in many planned homebirth narratives. For low-income women who gave birth in public sector clinics and hospitals, medical measurements were also an important interpretive framing device for making birth stories. However, these women were often denied biomedical and clockwork measurements by health care personnel in public sector birth settings. Authoritative ownership of the clockwork script and the right to interpret and regulate bodies according to its norms/measurements were firmly in the hands of health care workers in these instances. Within the sociomaterial space of the hospital or clinic, clockwork birth materialized different kinds of bodies and different opportunities for agency than in homebirth assemblages. In medicalized birth assemblages, women were often not granted epistemic opportunity to position their embodied experiences in relation to the clockwork narrative. At the same time, references to clocktime and biomedical measurements (or the lack of such measurements) were strong features of their tellings.

A key characteristic of clockwork birth was the telling of a formulaic birth story in which the embodied experience of labor/birth often disappeared. Preambles or 'run-ups' to labor/birth often became the focus of narrative drama rather than the psychofleshy birth experience itself. As a result, the preamble was often the most elaborated part of women's clockwork stories. Middle-class women (across a range of modes of birth) often told humorous and dramatic preambles, many of which involved some kind of complication, 'trouble' or comic subplots. For example, Stephanie told her homebirth story with a lengthy preamble, involving a series of dilemmas that emanated from the breeched position of her baby in the late stages of pregnancy. Her story began as follows (for an explanation of transcription notation please see Appendix 2):

Rachelle: Well, how was the birth? What happened?
Stephanie: *All right well*, um (★), there was, there was quite, there was quite a run-up to the actual birth itself (R: okay) cause we obviously had our heart set on birthing at home, um, and I carried very, very big, a lot of amniotic fluid (R: yes) and he [baby] was very mobile in the womb, in uterus, and he was either lying *transverse* (R: okay) *or* eventually settled um in a breech position (R: oh no) we were horrified.

(White, planned homebirth)

Stephanie's preamble then proceeded as a series of mini-stories involving several dramatic visits to various experts (including an acupuncturist) to try and get the baby turned into a conventional birthing position, dealing with the dilemmas of whether to still birth at home or not and practicing natural methods of inducing labor (i.e. castor oil and lovemaking). Once 'real' labor was diagnosed in her story, which she attributes to clear embodied knowing ("and I knew um") but that was also clearly ascertained by timing the contractions ("he [husband] was timing"), the clockwork birth recipe hums along in a predictable fashion. The midwife is called, there are vaginal examinations, her birthing body is plotted in centimeters ("I was five centimeters dilated"), labor progresses appropriately, the waters are broken and the baby is birthed in a matter-of-fact manner devoid of narrative detail. Stephanie tells the moment of birth as follows: "I sat on his [husband's] legs and at ten to one he was born, um." She then ends the story, "and that was that" with no details on what the moment of birth felt like, the delivery of the after-birth and any other messy, bloody or fleshy details erased. The birth event itself is reproduced as banal and routine. The psychofleshy experience of labor and birth as lived from Stephanie's perspective is thus largely muted and absent from the clockwork telling.

When enacting a clockwork script, low-income women told labor/birth as a series of clocktime happenings over which they had little to no control. Laboring/birthing bodies materialized as objects to be measured by authoritative others and were inscribed with centimeters and clocktime codes. For example:

Rachelle:	Can you tell me what happened from beginning to end? Basically your story of the birth?
Bonita:	I . . . the pain of course, and we went in [to the Maternal Obstetric Unit (MOU)], they examined me (*) and um we went in, they kept me, I was one and a half centimeters open so they kept me there and um after a few hours then they snipped my water (R: okay, okay).
Rachelle:	How many hours?
Bonita:	I (*) I was seven uuh (*) after five hours.
Rachelle:	Five hours? Okay.
Bonita:	Then they snipped my water because the pain was too bad, I couldn't stand it anymore, then they broke my water, then two hours after they snipped my water (R: hmm) then she came.

(Black, low-income, MOU birth)

This extract exemplifies the initial sparse and formulaic efforts of many women to narrate the psychofleshy birth experience. Some women went on to tell multivocal narratives that wove clockwork tellings with more complex fleshy stories of power, agency and embodied subjectivity (see Chapter 6). Others stuck to sparse and passive clockwork storylines in which they disappeared as active agents. In biomedical birth assemblages, particularly in public sector settings, clockwork stories were marked, not only by externally derived medical measurements, but also by the dominance of medical others as central agents of the birth event. As opposed to homebirth stories in which women themselves were often in control of reading and managing the laboring body, in the clockwork narratives of low-income women birthing in public sector settings, measurements, bodily signs and progress were medically managed, interpreted and controlled via interventions, medical instructions and direct orders. For example:

Nandipha:	I went to the, to the labor ward and then they checked me and they said that I am, I am three centimeters, so I should wait for a couple of hours **and then** it was around six (*) they said I must go to the, the bed (. . .) I slept there to, to wait for the hours.

(Black, low-income, MOU birth)

Celeste:	I was overdue (R: okay) that's why I went there [public hospital], um, the Tuesday I think about ten o'clock the night I got pains—**out of my own**—because I don't usually get pains, they give me (R: oh) and then it kept on till the next morning, the Wednesday morning about past ten and then I went, I was open about one to two centimeters and then **they** gave pains eight hours and it was four centimeters only (R: eight hours?) <u>again</u> eight hours and it was still four centimeters and then about 11 the Wednesday night <u>they decided</u> they are gonna caesar.

(Black, public hospital, emergency caesarean)

In these extracts, birth materializes as a process determined by medical outsiders. Decisions are made and pains are given without consultation. Birthing bodies become objects seemingly without capacities, feelings, knowledge or agency. It was typical in many low-income women's birth stories that medical others (the impersonal 'they') dominated birth stories. When women talked about the 'I,' it was often narrowly described in terms of outside definitions and prescriptions. Medicalized measurements often came to define the birthing woman—"I am three centimeters" (Nandipha) and "I was one and a half centimeters" (Bonita). Furthermore, when using the 'I voice,' it was often in terms of being ordered to do certain things—for example, "I should . . . I must" (Nandipha). In the extract from Bonita's story (see page 55), the generic "they" are the active actors in her birth experience, with little room available for her own feelings, sensations or psycho-fleshy experience. In the stories of many sociomaterially marginalized women, the labor experience was told as 'matter-of-fact,' filled with blank scenes of waiting and pain, in which the birthing woman was almost an incidental or absent character.

Abigail: Okay, the pains began the Sunday <u>night</u>, they kept me awake, then in the morning about (*) seven o'clock my sister-in-law came, then she asked if she must get transport and I said yes, okay, she went to get transport and then I went to X [MOU] then when I got to X [MOU] (*) then they examined me and said they were going to keep me because I was one centimeter open (R: okay) that was the morning, then the time went on there at X [MOU], they kept examining, went back to the labor ward (short laugh) the whole time until quarter past five #

Rachelle: In the evening?

Abigail: Yes, and then she was born,

(Black, low-income, MOU birth)

Bronwyn: Okay, it was the Saturday morning um half past three when I started having cramps (R: okay) I thought it was normal cause I normally have those cramps but then it started getting worse, then I went to go and wake my mommy up (*) and then she phoned my brother-in-law so we left here [home] at about half past four—I can't remember (both laugh) then we went to X [public hospital] yes, I lay there on that bed there— what do you call it—there where they examine you, I went there and I lay there for an hour, then I went to the labor ward (**) and I was in labor for about 45 minutes and then she was born yes (both laugh).

(Black, low-income, public hospital birth)

In the above extracts, birth is directed and managed by outside medical others. Labor and birth emerge in these tellings as banal, mechanical, passive and disembodied. The bodily experience of labor and birth is muted to such an extent that birth materializes as an unremarkable and mundane event. Furthermore, in these extracts, birthing women become almost invisible characters in the birth drama.

The clockwork narrative typically produced a series of gaps and omissions in which birth was either narrated as an abbreviated string of clichés (i.e. home-birthers) or a disembodied process dictated by medical authority figures. In both cases, the pulsating, visceral, embodied experience of labor and birth was muted. For example, consider Jeannie's account of her homebirth:

Rachelle: How <u>was</u> that birth? [First birth]
Jeannie: It went on very long, I mean I started with contractions, mild contrac-tions at like ten o'clock the Wednesday night (R: okay) *and* (★) I went in on the Thursday morning to Lily [midwife] and I said "{*I think I'm in labor*}, I haven't been able to sleep the whole night, something weird is going on, the dog has <u>not</u> left my side" (both laugh) and she said, "Well, you're smiling and you're walking in here, I'm not sure you are in labor. Let's have a look" and I was about one or two centimeters dilated so she said, "Okay, go home, when things get a little bit more hectic, phone me, otherwise I'll come in at about four or five o'clock and see how you're doing" so I didn't phone her cause everything was pretty much the same, by the time she came in, I think I was about, maybe about four centimeters dilated, but then we waiting like that until about eight o'clock at night and absolutely nothing changed, so eventually she broke the waters and then, then it started happening, ja [yes], and he came about quarter past midnight.

(White, planned homebirth)

What is missing here? Birth is told in relation to the clock and number of centim-eters dilated; there is a (comic) preamble, a series of measurements, the breaking of the waters and the story ends abruptly with the matter-of-fact statement "and he came about quarter past midnight." Any sense of the emotional and embodied experience of birth disappears in this telling. When asked to narrate a birth story, I found that many women responded initially with these kinds of abbreviated, matter-of-fact clockwork stories. This was true of women giving birth within different birth assemblages (e.g. private, public, homebirth) and across race/class divisions.

Abbreviated, sanitized, clockwork birth stories are recipes for telling birth that are embedded in biomedical ontologies. Often they function as a routine narrative recipe for how one goes about telling birth to friends and family—that is: give the outlines, plot the story in clocktime and leave out the messy, 'inappropriate' and bodily emotional details of labor and birth. This is perhaps why some women, pregnant for the first time, speak of a "vow of silence" (Cusk, 2001, p.18) about birth in which birth preparation literature and other women avoid telling them what birth is really like. As Angela (pregnant for the first time) lamented in a pre-birth interview, "no one *really* <u>tells you</u>, like <u>really</u> tells you the nitty-gritty (. . .) they all sort of gloss over it." Clockwork narratives thus function as cultur-ally appropriate, polite forms of birth storytelling because they omit the blood, pain, mess and emotional intensity of the labor/birth experience and tell birth as a linear and neatly packaged event (see Pollock, 1999). At the same time, they are framed within biomedical ontologies of birth, materializing birth as a linear, mechanical process and erasing the pulsating and paining corporeality of birthing. Furthermore, as I argue in the following section, these medicalized narratives did not just function as external frameworks but became materialized as part of women's ontological experiences of birth.

It must be noted that the clockwork narrative, with its ideal of linearity and coherence, was also entangled in the 'research assemblage' (Fox & Alldred, 2017) constituting the study. A linear clockwork script emerged as a narrative imperative that often framed birth interviews. For example, consider the following exchange:

Rachelle: Okay, what happened from beginning to end with the birth?
Erin: Okay, from the start? (R: yes) from the start, well she [baby] arrived one day before her due date (*) uh, her due date was Tuesday the 23rd and she was born at four o'clock in the morning on Monday the 22nd.

(White, planned homebirth)

Without being aware of this at the time, my narrative invitation was already framed within a linear logic and inadvertently might have encouraged women to tell coherent clockwork-like stories. As interviewer, I sometimes felt overwhelmed when women deviated from coherent linear ways of telling and often tried to bring them back to coherence by asking, 'so when did that happen?' As a result, clockwork narratives of birth were *co-constructions* that emerged between myself (as interviewer) and the woman telling the birth story.

Decoding the birthing body

A biomedical ontology, diffracted in/through the narrative script of clockwork birth, became part of women's stories and bodily experiences of birth. I argue that clockwork birth was not 'just' a narrative that represented women's 'real-life' experiences but that it was an intra-acting force and frame already operating within birth assemblages. The narrative script/recipe of clockwork birth intra-acted with other sociomaterial components of birth assemblages (space-location, institutional dynamics, class privilege/marginality, physiologies) to materialize bodies, stories and experiences differently. Across differings however, a clockwork vocabulary and script worked transversally to mute psychofleshy experiences of birth. At the same time, while constraining and disciplining storytelling and birthing bodies, the clockwork script was paradoxically used by some women as a mode of sensemaking, which provided a sense of control in relation to the fleshy materiality and unpredictability of the birthing body. Opportunities to use the clockwork script to enable forms of agency materialized predominantly in privileged birth assemblages (and particularly in homebirth settings).

Importantly (and somewhat ironically), the biomedical clockwork script gave some of the women interviewed a language with which to 'read' the birthing body and make the labor/birth process intelligible. Furthermore, in providing a formula and linear recipe, the clockwork script helped some women to manage the unpredictable birth process, make decisions and enabled them to construct ambiguous forms of agency. Different kinds of decisional dilemmas were enacted within different assemblages. For middle-class homebirthers, deciding when 'real' labor had kicked in and when to call the midwife were key moments. For low-income women, deciding when to go to the public health care clinic or hospital was narrated as central. Women needed to be able to 'read' or decipher the laboring body in order to make these decisions. Middle-class women who gave birth at home enjoyed the privilege of being able to call for medical help (i.e. a private midwife) as soon as they wanted to, while low-income women faced a series of hurdles in accessing health care that put them and their babies at risk. As a result, the narratives of low-income and middle-class women differed in terms of what kind of decision-making needed to be made during labor. For middle-class women, the dilemma of 'Is it or isn't it real labor?' dominated storytelling, while for women accessing public services, the relevant question became, 'Will I be admitted into health care services?'

Is it or isn't it 'real labor'?

Homebirthers were invested in using the clockwork narrative as a way of reading bodies and often engaged in a lot of 'discursive work' in order to make their birthing bodies conform to clockwork parameters. As a result, deciding *if and when* labor had truly started was a key dilemma that many middle-class homebirthers narrated in their narrative preambles. The question, 'Is it or isn't it?' 'real labor,' has been found by other studies to be an important narrative moment in middle-class women's birth stories, regardless of mode of childbirth (Akrich & Pasveer, 2004). In order to effectively invoke a clockwork script, one needs to be able to differentiate between 'real' labor and 'false' labor so that the clock can start ticking at the right time. The ability to accurately diagnose 'real labor' is thus necessary to maintain the integrity of a clockwork narrative. 'Real labor' was defined by women according to medical norms. In their narratives, homebirthers worked hard to fit their experiences into the clockwork script, with the 'real birth' only defined as kicking in with the diagnosis of labor according to clockwork logic. Thus, for Jane, "suddenly it was labor" because "the contractions were regular" coming "about 2/3 minutes apart and lasting about 40 seconds." Everything else she talked about before this, namely days of irregular contractions, feeling irritable and emotional, is swiftly dismissed as irrelevant. Homebirthing women used various terms to refer to the fuzzy, irregular period that was not 'real labor' according to medicalized clockwork norms. These terms included: "silly labor" (Jolene), "practice contractions" (Erin) and "false labor" (Sam). In efforts to make narrative coherence out of the fleshy birth experience, certain details were sometimes omitted in order to fit clockwork protocol. For example, Jolene told me, in her initial clockwork story that, "I had a contraction and that was that" signalling a clear, unambiguous starting point for 'real labor.' However, later on in her extended telling, she contradicted this version, hinting at a far more nebulous process of trying to decipher her laboring body:

Jenny: I was just trying to check that I was like definitely in labor (laughs) don't wanna phone her [midwife] and she comes all the way out here on a Sunday morning (laughs) (. . .) it's difficult to assess where labor actually, <u>where</u> you can sort of define cause you get silly labor where it's, like mild contractions every now and then.

(White, planned homebirth)

For many homebirthers, the fuzzy, vague and erratic stirrings of the emerging materiality of the 'body-in-labor' (Akrich & Pasveer, 2004) was challenging and frustrating. They wanted to 'read' this body and make it fit into a coherent clockwork script. Irregular contractions, unreadable signs of labor and periods of waiting for the process of labor to begin were thus often experienced as frustrating for middle-class women and their partners/family. For example:

Lizette: So we did that [had the midwife do a stretch and sweep], and then it was quite a weird experience then because then, um, you're kind of *really* in that waiting for something to happen (R: hmm) and little contractions did start happening then on the Thursday but it kept dying off, dying away (. . .) then we went to X's house where everything was gonna happen, and then we basically spent the Easter weekend, um, with like contractions coming and going and nothing really strong and regular, and I was, I was actually quite fine with that whole process but waiting is a, quite a difficult thing, it's difficult for a woman, uuh, I don't know if it's difficult for women or it's difficult for their partners (laughs) you know who kind of want something to happen now.

(White, planned homebirth)

As middle-class homebirthing women approached their 'due dates,' a silent and unreadable pregnant body became, in some cases (such as Lizette above) in itself 'a dilemma.' The laboring body that does not fit clockwork protocol becomes a potentially unreadable problem. This shows the entanglements of cultural narrative scripts as expectations that are used to frame, negotiate and decipher fleshy experience. Narrative scripts are thus part of the becoming of particular birthing assemblages and intra-act with other sociomaterial forces/components. Thus, given a birth assemblage shaped in part by clockwork expectations, Lizette's body, which produces contractions that 'die off' and 'die away,' becomes a point of frustration. While some middle-class women were themselves impatient and restless waiting for 'real labor' to begin (i.e. Joni and Sam), others felt pressurized by those around them to conform to timetables and norms. For example, Maggie's friends/ family got annoyed with her when her baby was not born at the expected time.

Maggie: Everyday people would phone me, so everybody had this expectation of me, and it's almost like they got really angry with me, I had friends down from overseas who had left by the time he was born and they came down to be here, to see him and they were almost like pissed off with me because "Why don't you have this baby? (R laughs) if you were in hospital they would've *induced* you, you could have had it already."

(White, planned homebirth)

In Maggie's case, failing to conform to clockwork expectations of labor/birth and not performing birth 'on time' was punished, not by the medical establishment, but by friends and family. This indicates the extent to which a biomedical clock-work narrative of birth has colonized everyday framings and expectations about birth. This also needs to be understood in the context of the wider spread of neo-liberal idealizations of choice, individual agency and consumerism that privilege the ability to plot, plan and control bodily processes. The idea of waiting for the birth process to begin in its own time is thus in itself an anathema to a technocratic 'ideology of control' (Diamond, 1994) which assumes that the body and nature can and should be regulated.

Will I be admitted into health care services?

The dilemma of pinpointing the starting point of 'real labor' was less prominent in the stories of low-income women birthing in public sector settings. These women were often more concerned with the question of when to go to the clinic or report to health services. In public sector clinic settings in South Africa, laboring women are sometimes turned away from health services if they are judged to be in the early stages of labor. Given that many of these women struggle to pay for transport to public health clinics, many literally cannot afford to be turned away from health services. They thus have to negotiate the tricky dilemma of reading their laboring bodies to decide if/when labor has advanced 'far enough' to gain legitimate admission to health care services. Low-income women do not have the luxury afforded to privileged South African women who were able to seek medical assistance as soon as desired. Many of these women described laboring at home for substantial periods of time, having contractions for hours or days until labor pains either became so bad that they "couldn't take it anymore" (Fadwah) or their waters broke. Some first-time birthers, despite laboring for hours at home before going in to the local clinic, were still turned away from health services and told they were not ready to be admitted because they were only in the early stages of labor. For example, Shiyaam labored at home for several hours before going in to the clinic because she thought her water had broken:

Shiyaam: And then I went to the hospital but when I got there then they said I was only <u>one</u> <u>centimeter</u> (R: oh okay) then they sent me back home.

(Black, low-income, MOU birth)

Similarly, first-time birther Fadwah, had pains for two days before going in to the local clinic. On examination, she was told that she was one centimeter dilated and given the choice of staying at the clinic or going back home. She decided to return home to continue laboring there. Her labor at home is narrated as a lengthy and dramatic experience in which, "the pains got worse and worse and worse" and her waters broke. At around this point she tells of turning to clockwork measurements to try and decode the laboring body, saying, "I timed my pains, it was four to five minutes (★) away from each other." Labor continued at home and she later passed blood and started to feel the urge to push. In her story, Fadwah only decides to return to the local clinic when she, "couldn't take it [pain] anymore."

In public sector birth assemblages in South Africa, a set of intra-acting forces, structures and sociomaterial relations result in the materialization of particular norms concerning when laboring women should present at health care services. These norms differ from the norms in middle-class, private sector birth assemblages. In medical birth assemblages shaped by privilege, women are encouraged to go to the hospital as soon as they think 'real labor' has begun and are not likely to be turned away from health services in the early stages of labor. The biomedical clockwork narrative is thus not homogenous or universal but materializes differently, producing different kinds of bodies and experiences according to sociomaterial locations. Medicalized birth, as a series of enactments, norms and sociomaterialities, thus operated according to a different logic for women in under-resourced public sector contexts in South Africa. Women were often disallowed from following the recipe steps outlined in the idealized (middle-class) medical clockwork script and described being sent away from health services in early labor. Some women were told by health care workers when they got to the clinic that they were not in labor and were sent home. Some women gave birth soon after being turned away from clinic services. For example:

Sharon: They [nurses] told me I was very far away from giving birth (★★) but then they said I must go home because (★) they said that I was still too far away from giving birth, but I gave birth that same night—then I got the child (R: okay) the same day that they told me it's not my time yet (★) but that same day I gave birth.

(Black, low-income, MOU birth)

While some low-income women timed their contractions, using clockwork measurements as a way of trying to decode the laboring body, others relied heavily on the advice of more experienced women relatives (mothers, aunts, sisters) in order to assess when they were in 'advanced' labor and it was time to go to health services. These relatives usually advised women to wait as long as possible before going to the clinic. For example, according to Jade, the advice from her aunt was that, "we must hang on a bit until my water broke (. . .) or they're gonna send me home." This meant that Jade waited for more than 12 hours before going to the MOU. Some low-income women miscalculated the progression of their labors, with the result that three women gave birth without a skilled caregiver and outside of health services. One baby was born at home with no caregiver and two were born in-transit to medical services (one was born in a mini-bus taxi and one baby was born in the yard of the local clinic). The network of biomedical power relations in the 'birth assemblage' for poor women thus did not always operate via heightened surveillance and medical interventions (see Chapter 4). Instead, the bodies and lives of poor women and their infants were not always prioritized at the level of everyday, local relations in public clinic health care settings, pointing to classed and racialized differings in the operation of biomedical power (Rabinow & Rose, 2006) on/through the bodies of poor, black women and middle-class women in the South African context.

Access to the clockwork medical script was thus not easily or automatically obtained by low-income women birthing in the public sector. Nurses served as gate-keepers who sometimes sent women home and refused them entry into clinics and biomedical scripts. The normative, idealized medical script was thus often rewritten in public sector clinic settings, with some laboring women constructed only as 'legitimate patients' if they were judged to be in advanced labor. The admission process materialized as unpredictable. It is also possible that some women were denied admittance due to space constraints in particular health care facilities (although this was not mentioned in women's narratives). One woman described being initially refused treatment at the local health care clinic, for reasons that were never clarified. For example:

Chumisa: The pains start to be strong, then I, my mom organized transport and then I go to the, to the midwife hospital, then when I arrived there, the nurses were, was not able to, to take care of me because they said I must wait (★★) outside the door ↑then they close the door↑, they say they (★★) are attending another patient #

Rachelle: So they wouldn't let you in?

Chumisa: They didn't even let me in, they said I must wait there, I wait there outside more than 30 minutes (★★) I arrived there I think (★) eight o'clock then they start to assist me I think at nine, twenty to nine.

(Black, low-income, MOU birth)

Medical attention was thus not always forthcoming when poor women presented themselves at health services. The clockwork script, as idealized biomedical recipe, was often unattainable because of class-based inequalities, structural impediments and differential patterns of biomedical power. Women were often left to their own devices, either sent away from health services or (as I will show in the following section) ignored and not monitored in clinic settings. While surveillance, monitoring and risk are key elements of the biomedicalization of birth in middle-class and privileged contexts, it is clear that biomedicalization does not operate upon poor women's bodies in the same way as those from the middle classes or residing in the Global North. According to Lupton (1997, p. 99), "The central strategies of disciplinary power are observation, examination, measurement and the comparison of individuals against an established norm, bringing them into a field of visibility."

The narratives of poor women suggest that, in the context of birth, the operation of 'disciplinary strategies' or concrete enactments of biomedical ontologies (i.e. measuring and monitoring) differ according to sociomaterial position. Poor black women's bodies often fall outside the gaze, are marginalized from the "field of visibility" (p. 99) and sometimes denied access to monitoring. As a result, many are left to negotiate labor (at home or in the clinic) without a great deal of intervention or 'medicalization.' While they rarely used the term in their narratives, low-income women more often than not succeeded at having 'natural births' and in some cases, what has been referred to as 'freebirths' (see Feeley et al., 2015). Their stories, however, reveal the degree to which 'natural childbirth' and 'freebirth' are middle-class terms embedded in sociomaterial positions of privilege. Moreover, their stories suggest that the idea of 'natural childbirth' or 'freebirth' as a triumph of women's empowerment and bodily power over medicalization is located in a narrow middle-class perspective that often ignores the privileges that shape and enable these discourses and practices. Middle-class ideals of 'natural birthing' are based on (the often unacknowledged and assumed) access to prompt medical attention if/when necessary. Poorer women do not always have the luxury of prompt medical attention, with the result that they face risks and difficulties during 'natural birth' that middle-class women do not. Encouraging a normative situation in which women labor at home until pains are so bad that they 'can't take it anymore,' is risky and communicates structural disregard for women's health and their lives.

Gaining access to health services was thus constructed in low-income women's birth narratives as an important element of the birth story script. Women needed to interpret the laboring body in order to decide if labor was far enough progressed to gain legitimate admission into health facilities. Women used clockwork measurements and signs (i.e. timing of contractions, breaking of the waters) as well as physiological sensations (is the pain 'bad enough?') and the advice of more experienced family members, to make these decisions. Once women gained admission into health care services, the clockwork script as a repertoire of sensemaking was, however, still not automatically available to them. Both women from marginalized sociomaterial positions and middle-class women giving birth in private hospitals were not always afforded the luxury of making birth intelligible or meaningful via the clockwork script. At times, low-income women and middle-class women giving birth in private hospitals were not given access to the information that would enable them to construct embodied forms of agency in/through clocktime measurements.

Denied access to clockwork knowledge in medical settings

Most women that I spoke to articulated desire for medical information and monitoring during labor. While women in homebirth settings usually had full access to details regarding medical assessments from their midwives, this kind of information was not always available to women in hospital or clinic settings. For example, first-time birther Angela, who wanted to have a 'natural' birth at a local private hospital, was not given enough information about the progression of her own labor to be able to 'read' her body or find a grid within/against which to interpret her raw, bodily sensations. After being left almost completely alone for nearly seven hours, Angela eventually demanded that the hospital midwife 'does a check.'

Angela: Eventually I said to her [midwife], "You know, I don't know *what's* happening, can't you do a check <u>now</u>?"

(White, private hospital birth, emergency caesarean)

Without information about medical measurements and 'progress,' Angela was left feeling lost and without a way of negotiating or making sense of the corporeal labor process. In her birth story, which turns out to be something of a 'horror story' (Pollock, 1999), medical personnel repeatedly deny her the right to knowledge and information about her own labor/birth process. Unknown drugs are administered through an intravenous drip, machines and monitors deliver information that is not shared with her and she is never given a clear reason why she has to have an emergency caesarean section. In her own words, she is left 'traumatized' and bereft after the birth and filled with unanswered questions and doubts about what really happened. At the time of our second interview (three months post-birth), she had been diagnosed with postnatal depression and was on antidepressive medication.

Having medical information and details about labor withheld was common-place in the narratives of low-income women giving birth in public sector settings. Some poor women spoke strongly about their *desire* for monitoring and informa-tion. Being left alone, without monitoring and medical feedback was described as anxiety-provoking and distressing. Women laboring in public sector clinics, often *wanted* to be assessed and subject to the biomedical gaze. For example:

Wendy: ^^Nobody came^^ the pains got <u>stronger</u> and <u>stronger</u> and um (*) then I went to one sister and *asked* her like (**) "Won't she check me to see how *far* I am, how many centimeters I am?" and um then she said "No, um, does she, do I <u>want</u> one, one of them to get ***angry*** with me?" they are going to get **angry** and <u>scold</u> me if I now ask how many centimeters and that they must <u>check on me</u> (R laughs) (both laugh) and then <u>um</u> (*) ^^then I left it and then went back to the room^^ because I didn't want big trouble, then I left it and nobody checked me.

(Black, low-income, MOU labor, transferred to public hospital)

Wendy was upset by the treatment at the local MOU, saying, "It was not a good experience for me *there* (*) it was not at all good." She was clear that the experi-ence would have been improved if, "they maybe checked on me and told me every time how many centimeters I was." As it was, she was left stranded and stuck in a limbo space where she "did not know" what was happening. Wendy expressed her dissatisfaction with the lack of care and medical monitoring at the clinic: "I, I, I think it's, it's not actually right." Other women birthing in public sector contexts also hinted at a lack of information or monitoring as a problematic issue. For example:

Sanele: They [nurses] didn't check, they say (*) if *you* feel like the baby's coming you must <u>go</u> and (**) you must <u>go to the bed</u> (R: and then call?) Then you call for them, but they *didn't* say, they didn't give us the, the minutes.

(Black African, low-income, public clinic birth)

Constance: Then I *asked* that other girl, "Don't they come and check your thingies, how many centimeters you are open?" Then she said, "No, you must just wait till they come and say you are going to give birth" and that, and then you just give birth.

(Black, low-income, public clinic birth)

For most women, across race–class divides, it was important to have access to medical information about the progression of their labors so that they could construct some sense of control in the midst of a painful and often overwhelming bodily experience of birth. Women thus *used* medical measurements to negotiate the psychofleshy labor experience. This illustrates the entanglement of external metrics, technologies and fleshy sentience in the corpomaterial experience of birth. The birthing body is not simply a mechanical, biomedical object but is a lived intertwining involving complex psychofleshy negotiations of physiological and sociocultural forces, feelings and frames (see Leder, 1992). Bodily experiences of labor/birth were thus not separate from socioculture but inextricably entangled with ontological and narrative frames. Denying women medical information about their labors had affective consequences, resulting in feelings of disempowerment and anxiety during labor/birth. Furthermore, the lack of adequate monitoring and information ultimately sends messages that women are insignificant and unimportant and/or that they are too ignorant to need/understand information about their own bodies. Withholding information also bolsters hierarchical biomedical power relations and reiterates the idea that it is medical staff that hold authoritative power to define, manage and make sense of birth. In the words of Constance, "you must just wait till they come and say you are going to give birth and that, and then you just give birth." Birthing women become reduced, in these kinds of encounters, to passive and empty characters who wait on medical permission and instruction, and are then expected to "just give birth" like dehumanized, faceless body-machines.

Some low-income women took matters into their own hands and timed their own contractions to try and make sense of the embodied sensations of labor via clockwork measurements. For example, Gertrude and her husband were left completely alone during her labor and she received no monitoring. According to her story, she had only one vaginal examination during her labor and this occurred only when, "I screamed and I said that it was burning," just minutes before delivery. At this point, she was already fully dilated. Before this, Gertrude was left to her own devices to manage the pains and bodily challenges of labor. With her husband's help, she was, however, able to time contractions and find some way of interpreting the painful labor process. For example:

Rachelle: How was the pain?
Gertrude: The pain? They were light at first then afterwards they were bad, because I was five minutes apart (. . .)
Rachelle: Okay, so during that time you were actually timing?
Gertrude: *Yes,* then, then the pain was too bad (★) then he said it's now two minutes apart.
Rachelle: Who said?
Gertrude: My husband (. . .) yes, then he said it's now two minutes, it's no longer five minutes.

(Black, low-income, MOU birth)

Similarly, Sharon timed contractions herself, saying, "When I looked at my watch the pains that I got were almost every 20 minutes." Other women timed the pains while they were at home waiting to decide when to go into the clinic; according to Fadwah, "I timed the pains, it was four to five minutes (★) away from each other."

Most of the women interviewed said explicitly that they wanted access to information, not only about the progression of their labors, but about all aspects of the birth process. Not being given such information was a key ingredient of a dissatisfying birth experience. Being denied information about their own bodies left some women feeling like they were not full actors in their own birth experiences. Vanessa explained how she was sent, in an emergency ambulance from a local MOU to a public hospital, without any kind of explanation about what was wrong.

Rachelle: How did you feel when they sent you there? [public hospital]
Vanessa: Uh no, not nice, because I wasn't sure why, they don't explain, they just say, "The ambulance is going to fetch you, to go to X," they explain nothing, just he's coming to fetch you and then *off you go.*

(Black, low-income, MOU labor transferred to
public hospital for birth)

Women giving birth in public sector clinic settings were thus often either hardly monitored at all or not informed about medical measurements and the 'progress' of labor. As a result, the message communicated was that medical knowledge, expertise and birth itself, belongs to medical practitioners. Laboring women (as persons and lived bodies) became unimportant and incidental figures and the laboring/birthing body was framed as purely a biological entity to be probed and prodded for signs of deviance. Without explanation or information about what and why things were happening, some women were left unable to stitch the birth experience into a coherent and agentic narrative (i.e. Vanessa above). Ultimately, the stories of low-income women show that the clockwork narrative is rooted in a biomedical ontology of birth, which enacts medical practitioners and health care workers as experts and women as incidental characters in the birth drama. While homebirthers often managed to use the clockwork script as a frame to construct empowering forms of agency, women in medicalized settings were often denied this opportunity, experiencing medicalization in health care settings as a restriction on embodied agency and sensemaking.

Unruly bodies: when the clockwork body fails

While medical information was often withheld from low-income women in the public sector and middle-class women birthing in private hospitals, homebirthers were often able to use the clockwork script to enact ambiguous forms of agency. However, when the clockwork narrative imploded because the forceful materiality of laboring/birthing bodies failed to conform to the script, homebirthers experienced the power of this narrative as a normative biomedical ideal that disciplines unruly bodies. Interestingly, women's stories suggest that many participants went into the birth experience already armed with the clockwork story as interpretive device and expectation-related framework. Consider Mandy's story about her first homebirth, which failed to meet the expectations she held in relation to birth:

Mandy: I labored beautifully, I **loved** laboring, um (*) and then at, at about seven centimeteres I got into the bath and that was just amazing, and then I got stuck on nine centimeters, laboring hard and she [midwife] said okay she's going to break my water for me (. . .) and then obviously that gush brings the baby down even more and suddenly your contractions just come, um, and then the pain was too overwhelming for my body and I, I vomited in the birthing bath so I had to get out and um, so she said to me "Right, you're ten centimeters now"—now antenatal classes and all the books and all the teachings said at ten centimeters you get this, quote unquote "unbearable urge to bear down, nothing can stop this urge from coming and all you want to do is bear down and push"—that didn't happen, um, which I was waiting for, I thought, "okay right" cause friends of mine who had given birth a couple days earlier, this was also part of their story, they said "ooh, it was just overwhelming, you just had to squat and push you know."

(White, planned homebirth)

As typical in the clockwork narrative, Mandy plots her laboring body in relation to number of centimeters dilated, with normative measurements being used to mark her 'progress' through the birth experience. However, when the script fails and her body falls silent, failing to produce the expected 'urge to push' at ten centimeters, Mandy's birth comes undone—i.e. "I can't do this (. . .) I couldn't push." The 'textbook' story fails to materialize because her laboring body does not conform to expectations. She describes waiting for this part (the urge to push) of the script to happen, showing how the clockwork narrative (as sensemaking repertoire) can become knitted into women's own expectations and lived experiences of birth (Pollock, 1999). Without this script, Mandy is left with no meaningful "interpreta-tive framework" (Pollock, 1999, p. 131) within which to make birth and the fleshy material force of the birthing body intelligible. She is unable to construct a position as an embodied self (Akrich & Pasveer, 2004). As a result, the words used repeat-edly to describe her 'I' voice are passive and constrained and filled with a sense of being unable, unknowing and incapable: "I can't . . . I couldn't . . . I don't know." The fleshy birthing body enacts its own forceful agency during labor/birth that has to be read, negotiated and made sense of. The clockwork script functions as an important framing device that mediates body–self relations during labor/birth. When the script fails or is withheld, women are often left unable to construct forms of embodied agency. Similarly to Mandy, Jane narrated a first homebirth in which the clockwork narrative she was expecting failed to materialize. Jane spoke of hav-ing, "quite set expectations":

Jane: I thought if you're relaxed enough and if you've read enough and if you do everything right, you know, it won't hurt (both laugh) so I was really taken aback by the real actual (R: ferocity?) ja [yes], and I felt, I actually felt in it that I am doing everything wrong and I am being a complete failure.

(White, planned homebirth)

In Jane's description, we can see how the clockwork script can discipline women during labor/birth via the enactment of norms and regulatory ideals. It is also important to emphasize that the clockwork narrative is a variant of 'natural' or 'normal' birth, all of which are thoroughly embedded in biomedical frameworks. The concept of 'natural' birth is based on the writings of male medical practitioners such as Grantly Dick-Read and Ferdinand Lamaze, who postulated that labor and birth can (and should) be pain-free if women use the correct relaxation and breath-ing techniques (Dick-Read, 1933, 1963; Lamaze, 1958). In contrast to the ideals of clockwork or 'natural' birth, Jane experiences an erratic labor with irregular contractions in which she takes 19 hours to dilate to five centimeters. Furthermore, she experiences labor as extremely painful, which does not conform to her ideal-ized expectations framed in/through a 'natural birth' model. As a result, Jane is left feeling like "a complete failure."

Michelle also told a birth story in which the fleshy materiality of her laboring body exerted its own powerful agency and urgency, shattering her expectations about how her second homebirth would unfold. She started feeling contractions late in the evening and expected that (like her first birth) labor would take a long time to unfold. However, 30 minutes after she started to feel contractions she suddenly felt, "like a pushing feeling" and "really got a shock." The midwife was contacted and Michelle had to try and stop herself from pushing until she arrived. This period of waiting for the midwife while feeling the urge to push and bear down is described as intense, harrowing and frightening. According to Michelle, "I was actually very scared" and "it was *incredibly* intense (. . .) I was actually incredibly *scared* you know." The laboring body exerted its own powerful force/agency and Michelle could not cope. She explains:

Michelle: So when the contractions happened, you know they were intense ones, it was, it was *incredibly*, it was like I couldn't, I couldn't cope (R: ja) it just felt like this pain was just, I couldn't handle it.

(White, planned homebirth)

In Michelle's story, the fleshy laboring body has its own agency that does not always fit into clockwork norms and expectations. When the midwife tried to give her instructions at the time of pushing, the force of the body was more powerful: "I actually said my body can't stop now, it just has to do this (. . .) I just couldn't stop pushing." The force of the laboring body is sometimes overwhelming, leaving some women unable to construct forms of embodied agency and feeling disconnected from their bodies. This can happen even during unmedicated, non-interventionist, 'natural' labor at home. Thus, Michelle said she would have preferred more time or "a couple of more hours of labor (. . .) of <u>knowing</u> I was in labor maybe, of maybe having more of an awareness." According to Akrich and Pasveer (2004), there are two forms of bodily agency present in women's birth narratives, namely: the physiological, fleshy 'body-in-labor' and the 'embodied self.' Women's experiences of birth are told as a complex movement between these two forms of bodily agency and thus invariably involve duality. This duality is, however, not always alienating. Akrich and Pasveer (2004) suggest that positive experiences of birth depend on the construction of a meaningful resonance, relational dynamic or form of connection between fleshy body-in-labor and embodied self. Birth is experienced as alienating when women are unable to form such a relationship, "either because the body-in-labor is too present and takes over, or because it is absent" (p. 80). In Michelle's case, the fleshy, paining body is 'too present' and she is unable to forge any meaningful relationship between it and the 'I' voice (embodied self). The materiality of the laboring body thus has its own agency (Barad, 2007) that is forcefully felt by some women during birth as a shattering of the coherent self, expectations and sociocultural norms.

For most homebirthers, however, the clockwork script hummed along fairly easily as births unfolded, for the most part, in a 'textbook' fashion, without complication or major deviation (see Chapter 6 for an exploration of how this worked to subvert medical master narratives). As a result, many women were able to use the clockwork script to manage labor, construct forms of embodied agency and situate themselves positively in relation to the birth process.

Significantly, homebirthing midwives usually respected and recognized the embodied knowledge of women-in-labor. As a result, clockwork measurements could be used in conjunction with women's bodily sensations to construct forms of embodied agency. Clockwork measurements and monitoring techniques were often able to make the fleshy birthing body talk in a rational, orderly language, which was comforting to many women. Furthermore, plotting labor according to clockwork measurements enabled women to tell coherent and linear birth stories. Ironically, the medically derived clockwork story could thus be used to subversively reconstruct birth (in the private homebirth assemblage) as a normal and routine process that women's bodies are good at (see Chapter 6).

Summary

This chapter explored biomedical power as entangled with/in women's birth narratives. Far from being a totalizing, coherent and external force, medicalization was found to be intimately interwoven with/in the frames women used to make meaning about labor and birth. Women's stories suggest that in relation to birth, biomedicine is a form of power, "that extends throughout the depths of consciousness and bodies of the population" (Hardt & Negri, 2000, p. 24). As a result, an idealized medical narrative of birth, what I have termed, 'the clockwork narrative,' framed women's efforts to narrate and make sense of labor and birth. Importantly, women across race/class divides often *desired* a clockwork script as a way of reading, decoding and managing fleshy sensations and pain. If women were accorded epistemic opportunities to make sense of the psychofleshy labor/birth experience via clockwork measurements and information, they were often able to negotiate and enact forms of embodied agency. This shows the entanglement/s of medical ontologies and fleshy corporeality, disrupting any clear separation between biomedicine and physiological birth. It also suggests that efforts to demarcate the phenomenon of 'natural' or physiological labor/birth as separate from culture, medicine or technology, are misguided. At the same time as clockwork measurements enabled forms of embodied agency (particularly for homebirthers), the narrative also worked to produce laboring/birthing bodies as measurable objects and disciplined fleshy experiences. As a result, when women framed their experiences within this narrative script, the undecidability and psychofleshy complexities of labor/birth were often muted and erased. Biomedical power relations thus work intimately and relationally within birth assemblages, with unpredictable and ambiguous results. Women can be empowered or disempowered by biomedical information and scripts, depending on particular corpomaterial configurations.

Biomedical power relations did not operate in a singular or homogenous fashion but produced shifting ontologies and birthing bodies in different sociomaterial assemblages. The clockwork script was thus not equally available to all women. For example, in public sector contexts, women were often denied information about the progression of their labor (dilation centimeters), which left them feeling unsure, unsafe and anxious. Low-income women were also subject to particular medical norms within public sector clinic settings in which they were often only regarded as 'legitimate patients' if they were in advanced labor. Several women spoke about being sent home from health services early on in their labors, while others were familiar with the norms (either via previous experiences or the advice of family/friends) and tried to labor at home for as long as possible to avoid being sent away from clinic settings, usually until pains became too hard to bear anymore. The ideal clockwork narrative of birth, according to which women in early labor would access medical help as soon as possible, is shown to be predominantly a narrative of privilege. While middle-class women enjoy easy access to medical services, poor women have to struggle harder to access health care and be recognized as 'legitimate patients.' Biomedical power, embodied in measurements, practices and authoritative forms of expertise, was also more likely to materialize as a constricting, coercive and disempowering set of relations in medicalized assemblages, including private and public sector hospitals and clinics. Poverty, race and medicalization intra-acted in birth assemblages to result in fewer opportunities for clockwork agency in the narratives of low-income women birthing in the public maternity sector.

In privileged homebirth assemblages, women were often able to use the clockwork interpretive framework (via signs, measurements, norms and information provided by midwives) to decode the fleshy, laboring body and negotiate forms of embodied agency. At times, however, the force of the laboring body failed to conform to expectations and clockwork grids and normative storylines imploded. In such cases, women were left feeling shattered and struggled to construct positive forms of embodied agency. Biomedical power thus emerged as a relational force that intra-acted with sociomaterial location and fleshy physiology to produce unpredictable effects. At the same time, biomedical ways of framing birth and birthing bodies dominated women's stories.

This chapter suggests that biomedical power is intimately interwoven into the process of making birth narratives. Telling a birth story (even of homebirth), is largely dependent on using medicalized vocabularies of labor and birth. Similar to Sbisà (1996, p. 371), careful analysis showed that biomedical descriptions, norms and measurements, "constitute the basic vocabulary with the aid of which women imagine their forthcoming [birth] experience." Biomedical power is thus entangled with women's desires, experiences and expectations of birth, regardless of whether women birth at home or in medicalized settings. However, as an 'internalized technology of power,' biomedical power is not discrete and does not operate in isolation. Instead, it is thoroughly intersectional and material, intertwining with race, class, other modes of social marginalization, material institutions (public/private, clinic/hospital) and fleshy bodies, to construct diffractive 'lived realities' of birth.

4

RISKY BODIES

Over the last 40 years, biomedical risk has come to define experiences of pregnancy and birth, particularly in the Global North (Helen, 2004). The definition of birth as a medical event has dovetailed with a growing emphasis on risk and the belief that birth requires medical interventions, monitoring and biotechnology in order to be 'safe.' While birth has become safer than ever for women in the Global North, risk vocabularies have paradoxically intensified in these contexts (Lankshear, Ettore & Mason, 2005). The language of risk is embedded in the logic and practices of contemporary obstetrics and operates within a 'technico-scientific' model of risk in which expert and evidence-based knowledge, prediction and control is emphasized (Lupton, 1999a). 'Risk' in relation to birth thus predominantly means biomedical risk and incorporates a growing plethora of conditions, abnormalities, deviations and syndromes associated with conception, pregnancy, labor and birth. The dominance of risk discourse in maternity care protocols and birth management in Northern settings is widely accepted; even midwives have been found to be preoccupied with discourses of biomedical risk, surveillance and the dangers of birth (Lankshear, Ettore & Mason, 2005; Seibold et al., 2010; Scamell, 2011; Scamell & Alaszewski, 2012). Studies exploring pregnant women's constructions of risk in the Global North have also found that biomedical risk dominates women's talk about pregnancy and birth. For example, in a study of Australian women who gave birth in a range of contexts (at home, birth center and hospital), Possamai-Inesedy (2006) found that talk of biomedical risk suffused women's accounts, with little evidence of alternative constructions. Other studies have however found that 'risk' can mean different things to different women, depending on birth assemblages (Miller & Shriver, 2012; Chadwick & Foster, 2014). For example, studies have found that women who plan homebirths associate risk with being in the hospital and emphasize loss of control, agency and potential interventions as significant risks during hospital birth (Edwards & Murphy-Lawless, 2006; Lindgren et al., 2008; Viisainen, 2000). There has, however, been little research that has explored risk and birth beyond normative conceptualizations of biomedical risk.

Obstetrics increasingly operates through molecular (rather than overtly punitive) relations of power, which materialize as a range of disciplinary strategies, frames, techniques, authority relations and discourses (Arney, 1982). These biopolitical strategies and technologies resonate powerfully in the rhetoric and practices of 'risk politics' (see Rose, 2001). Risk politics in relation to birth does not, however, materialize in a homogenous fashion, but as I will show in this chapter, differs according to location, geopolitics and socioeconomics. Obstetrics is intertwined with bioeconomics and inseparable from the capitalization and commodification of medical expertise, technologies and interventions. Risk politics, bioeconomics and maternity care are thus complexly entangled and materialize as different kinds of 'risk economies' in relation to pregnancy/birth. Northern-based researchers often reproduce a singular, monolithic story about risk and birth and assume that the intensification of biomedical risk in relation to pregnancy/birth operates homogenously via increased surveillance and technocratic intervention. Potential differences in the materialization of biomedical risk and risk politics according to socioeconomics and geopolitics have not been widely explored. Problematically, studies of risk and birth have been overwhelmingly based on the perspectives of privileged women in the Global North. There has been little examination of risk and birth from the perspectives of marginalized women in the Global South. As a result, we know little about risk politics in these settings or how a framework of 'biomedical risk' might materialize differently in practices, norms and methods of managing pregnancy and birth. According to Olofsson et al. (2014, p. 419), there has been a broader failure in health and sociological research to acknowledge "the power dimensions of risk constructions." There have also been few studies exploring the ways in which socioeconomics and race impact on the logic/practices of biomedical modes of birth more broadly (see Bridges, 2011, as exception).

In this chapter, I extend the analysis of biomedical power begun in the previous chapter by exploring the different risk economies materializing in/through women's birth narratives. Importantly, I will show that enactments of risk differed according to sociomaterial positionings. When it comes to birth, risk politics are entangled with socioeconomics and differ according to race/class locations. While risk politics operated via the normative construction and negotiation of labor/birth as risky and biomedical interventions, expertise and monitoring as the route to safety during birth in privileged birth assemblages, in under-resourced and marginalized settings, the politics of risk and birth materialized differently. Far from being subject to increased monitoring and surveillance, low-income women were often subject to biomedical *invisibilization* during labor/birth in which they disappeared, were forgotten and disregarded, and fell outside of the medical gaze. Monitoring, machines and interventions were often missing and many women were left to labor alone with no medical assistance or pain relief. In addition to 'risks to life' stemming from a lack of biomedical care and monitoring, low-income women were also faced with 'risks to self' and dignity in public sector contexts. Thus, while the biomedical definition of birth as a risky event requiring medical care/intervention framed women's experiences and narratives of birth across diverse sociomaterialities, biomedical risk was enacted differently according to positions of privilege/marginalization.

While biomedical risk politics materialized differently across sociomaterialities, women's birth stories also enacted multiple forms of risk. The 'risky body' of birth was not singular. Risk in relation to birth was thus not only about biomedical risk. Women were also worried about other kinds of risks, notably the distinctive bodily risks posed by the corporeal vulnerability of the laboring/birthing body. Patriarchal constructions of women's reproductive bodies as abject, monstrous and disgusting (see Ussher, 2006; Chadwick & Foster, 2013) enacted a different form of 'risky body' in relation to birth and framed fears and anxieties among middle-class women. Losing privacy and bodily dignity during labor/birth were significant concerns for privileged women and shaped their birth choices. While privileged women worried about these risks, it was low-income women that experienced them. Poor women birthing in public sector contexts thus had to negotiate multiple 'risks to self' during birth, including: dehumanization, violence, loss of dignity and the absence of medical and supportive care. Exploring the diffractive meanings of risk in different risk economies shows that 'risk' is not one thing in relation to birth and that while biomedical understandings of risk frame the narratives of most women, there are also other (often silenced) risks that women negotiate in relation to birth. This chapter explores the multiple kinds of 'risky bodies' enacted in women's birth narratives. It also traces the emergence of different 'risk economies' according to sociomaterial positionings.

Biomedical risk economies: privilege, technocratic bodies and moral identities

> [T]here's too much uncertainty, there's too many variables.
> *(Hannalie, white, elective caesarean section)*

Giving birth in the technocratic, highly resourced, profit-driven, private health care sector in South Africa means being embedded in a biomedical risk economy in which pregnant women are highly monitored, usually have medical experts (obstetricians and gynaecologists) as primary caregivers and are likely to experience highly interventionist births. This is a risk economy shaped by privilege, profit, capitalization and technocracy. Unsurprisingly, middle-class women utilizing private sector services framed their talk about birth choices in relation to an overarching discourse of biomedical risk. This included women that chose to birth at home. Women differed, however, in their orientations towards medicalization and technocratic interventions. Those who chose elective caesareans thoroughly embraced technocratic birth and dominant understandings of biomedical risk while women planning homebirths drew on multiple and shifting definitions of risk, both contesting and confirming biomedical risk discourses.

Elective caesarean as a form of risk management

Women who chose elective caesareans regarded birth as *essentially* risky. Choosing an elective caesarean section was constructed as a form of risk management. In line with a technico-scientific model of risk, obstetric risks in the form of abnormalities and complications were seen as controllable or avoidable with expert obstetric knowledge and maximum degrees of technocratic monitoring and intervention. All of the women who chose caesarean sections consulted specialist obstetricians and gynaecologists during pregnancy and had an ultrasound at every visit to their medical doctor. Some also had additional monitoring at a 'foetal assessment center' and two had amniocentesis testing. When talking about their birth choice, women invariably constructed caesarean section as a 'safer choice' than vaginal birth. The physiological process of 'natural' birth was seen as inherently risky, unpredictable and dangerous. According to Hannalie, "there's too much uncertainty, there's too many variables." The caesarean section was seen as the best way to deal with the uncertainties posed by the laboring/birthing body and guarantee a positive outcome. In these stories, technology was constructed as the solution to risk and never seen as potentially iatrogenic. Women choosing caesareans thus overwhelmingly used a normative vocabulary of biomedical risk to frame and justify their birth choices. For Hannalie, biomedical technology was the best way to manage, "too many things that can go wrong." For example:

Hannalie: She [sister–in–law] had a normal birth the first time and then the second time the baby was overdue two weeks, and only the morning when they did the induction and they put the heart monitor on, did they realize that this baby has been in distress because there's no amniotic fluid left and then they realized if they don't take the baby out now, it's not going to survive, and then I ask myself now what would have happened if they didn't, you know, if they didn't put the monitor on? You know, so I dunno, I think these things should be controlled, it's, it's, there's just too many things that can go wrong.

(White, middle-class)

Birth via caesarean section was constructed as professional, safe, modern and predictable whereas the bodily process of labor/birth was regarded as unpredictable and unsafe. For example:

Lola: She [gynaecologist] can tell me exactly what happens with a caesar, but for normal birth, you never know, you're never sure exactly what's going to happen.

(White, middle-class)

Janine: You dunno how long it's [natural birth] gonna last, you dunno if you're gonna end up with a caesar in any case (. . .) so (*) ja, you just don't (*) know what, what's gonna happen (R: okay).

(White, middle-class)

These extracts show an investment in a biomedical approach to birth, which promises prediction and control, reproduces technocratic birth as safe birth and enacts the birthing body as essentially unsafe and risky. An elective caesarean section was seen as the ultimate enactment of technico-science's ability to conquer risk and unpredictability. Thus, according to Hannalie, "why would you have a normal birth if you can have a caesarean section." Biomedical modes of birth, particularly caesarean sections, were regarded by these women as part of a narrative of medical progress. According to Caroline, "we've *progressed* with modern medicine (. . .) for me, it's a choice that makes sense to me, you know we've progressed." Similarly, Hannalie likened the progression in techniques relating to heart surgery to modern forms of surgical birth.

Hannalie: I mean, there (*) medical procedures have advanced so much today, if you look at the way they do a heart operation, they do it differently to the way they did it ten years ago (R: hmm). Why would you then go the normal route, if you, why would you go the old route of a heart operation, if you can go the new route? Why would you have a normal birth if you can have a caesarean section?

(White, middle-class)

Biomedical risk economies were not only shaped by socioeconomics and the valorization of technoscience but were also enacted in narratives as a form of moral politics. According to Rabinow and Rose (2006, p. 197), biopower involves the following elements: truth discourses, authorities, "strategies for intervention" and modes of subjectification in which individuals, "are brought to work on themselves." Obstetric power operates via all of these elements in biomedical risk economies, galvanising moral enactments in the name of potential 'risks to life' (usually the unborn baby). The association between moral values and beliefs about the protection of life and biomedical technocracy means that obstetric medicine is sanctioned with ensuring the conception and safe delivery of legitimate and valuable forms of life (i.e. 'normal' without abnormalities). As a result, preventing or eliminating 'risk/s to life' becomes a central expectation of obstetric medicine. It is not surprising, given that obstetric medicine and technology have become the social guardians of (legitimate) conception and life, that many pregnant women feel compelled to seek and enact 'practices of the self' that reiterate medicalized forms of biopower. The capacity to engage in 'practices of the self' that reiterate and perform mothering as a form of moral identity is produced most powerfully within privileged socioeconomic risk assemblages. As a result, choices about birth become moral dilemmas for many middle-class women in which they have to balance the 'risk to life' posed by birth with their own desires and truth frameworks. For women choosing caesareans, eliminating the unpredictable process of labor and birth and electing to have a surgical delivery, meant less 'risk to life' and ensured safety. According to Caroline, "there's less risk in a caesar nowadays" and for Hannalie, "there's just too many things that can go wrong" with vaginal birth. Furthermore, as Sarah explained:

Sarah: I just think that, because of once again, the unpredictability of it [birth], um, you don't know if somethings gonna go wrong and you dunno how quickly you're going to need <u>to act</u> if something goes wrong and why put your baby and yourself at risk like that?

(White, middle-class)

The widespread belief that safe birth equals birth in a biomedical setting with available technologies and interventions means that women choosing to give birth at home face particular challenges to their moral identities as a result of their birth choices. As a result, these women had to find ways of challenging biomedical definitions of birth while simultaneously protecting the ethics of the choice to birth outside the normative medical system.

Risk, homebirth and the power of 'what if . . . ?'

While women choosing caesareans were firmly invested in a normative biomedical risk economy, women planning homebirths were positioned more ambiguously in relation to biomedical questions surrounding birth and potential 'risks to life.' While valorizing an alternative model of birth, "spoken from a feminine subjectivity" (Young, 1990a, p. 193), in which bodily knowing, intuition, 'nature' and the spiritual realm were regarded as legitimate forms of knowing and being, homebirthers were nonetheless also faced with having to take up an ethical position vis-à-vis biomedical discourses of risk. They were caught in an ethical dilemma between wanting to affirm women's bodily capabilities and not wanting to take undue risks that might have life/death consequences. As a result, although 37-year-old Stephanie felt that, "I had a natural capacity to do this thing" [give birth], the power of the anxiety-provoking and biomedical risk-infused 'what if . . . ?' question continued to haunt her narrative. She admitted that her belief in her 'woman's capacity' was constantly challenged by the intrusion of biomedical risk discourse which appeared in the form of 'what if. . .?' questions.

Stephanie: It [decision to birth at home] was very challenged by, then I was 37 and first birth, just literally um culturally that negativity, that, that um challenged my confidence quite often, I would feel, "Am I doing the right thing?," "What if something goes wrong?" you know, how can I homebirth and then something goes wrong?

(White, middle-class)

Even after an uneventful first birth at home, Stephanie was still plagued by these risk-infused questions at the time of our conversation (which was a couple of weeks before she was due to have her second baby at home). Stephanie's account demonstrates how homebirthing women are ambiguously positioned in a biomedical risk economy. While attempting to subvert the authoritative power of biomedicine they are nonetheless 'affected' by its 'truths,' which generate anxiety, doubt and the loss of bodily confidence. Thus, while she had chosen to go without all medical technology in her first pregnancy (including ultrasound sonography), Stephanie decided in her second pregnancy that technology, "has a place" because of anxiety over her age, having twins and/or a baby with an abnormality.

Stephanie: I mean this time round when we had huge angst about twins, we went for scans, you need to know, I mean it's a huge economic thing, and um, being gradually worn down by nausea and feeling, "Am I going to do this?" and "I'm 42 this year and what if this is a Down's Syndrome baby?" "What if? What if? What if?" I went for an 18-week scan which was fascinating, absolutely fascinating, once I gave over to it you know, this has a place (. . .) um, to know whether there was abnormality, that we needed to be aware of and to prepare ourselves, it really has a place.

(White, middle-class)

Homebirthers were thus not purely located in a space of resistance against vocabularies of biomedical risk and technological interventions. Women were keenly aware of the cultural perceptions surrounding homebirth as a risky and dangerous practice and had to negotiate being branded as 'risk-takers' by friends and family. For example:

Michelle: I think she [friend] thought I was taking a terrible chance and it was a very risky thing to do and she'd had a friend in X who'd had a very bad homebirth experience where the baby actually passed away so I think it [reaction] was very mixed, people would say I'm very irresponsible, just thinking of my needs as opposed to what the baby would need and "What happens in X if there's an emergency? And how you're going to get to the hospital?" and um, and I would just quote statistics.

(White, middle-class)

Despite negative responses from some of her friends and the ever-present 'what if . . . ?' risk-infused questions that surrounded the choice to birth at home, for Michelle the risks of homebirth paled in comparison to the "the idea of being cut open." Other women had to deal with being thought "crazy" (Lizette) by those around them for planning a homebirth. However, these women feared the risks of hospital birth (indignity, exposure, medical interventions) more than the risks of birth at home.

At the same time, the decision to birth at home was also premised on the assumption that biomedical technology and intervention would be accessible and available if needed. All of the middle-class homebirthers made it clear in their stories that they would make full use of medical expertise and technology if it became necessary. They thus regularly made disclaimers such as, "but one needs to have some form of back-up" and "look, if I need to go to hospital I will, I'm not going to be stupid about it" (Angela). According to Cindy: "you're not ill when you're pregnant, you know, unless of course there's an emergency and then you thank god for medical intervention." While some of these women rejected all forms of testing and technology during pregnancy (i.e. Angela), others consulted extra specialists in sonography and had '3D' ultrasounds (i.e. Anke). Those women that rejected pregnancy testing and ultrasound monitoring were clear that they regarded these procedures as themselves 'risky.' For example, according to Angela, the long-term consequences of using sonography are not known, making it a risky practice.

> Angela: I think, you know, I mean what am I going to do if there is something wrong? And I think that the more one interferes the more likely that there is damage in the baby, you know, they say it's [ultrasound technology] linked to remedial difficulties and they don't actually know, I mean scanning hasn't been around for that long, they don't know the side effects.
>
> *(White, upper class)*

Angela subverts normative biomedical risk discourse in this extract, producing an alternative enactment of medical experts as unknowing and biomedical technology as dangerous and risky. Other women also questioned the legitimacy of medical technology and indicated a lack of trust in obstetric tests. For example, Jane refused to have more ultrasounds done after her (only) scan at 22 weeks because she felt they created unnecessary complications:

> Jane: I don't have scans at 36 weeks because then they start telling you, "Oh your baby's so big and your baby's this and your baby's that" and I'm like—"No, thank you."
>
> *(White, middle-classs)*

Middle-class women choosing to birth at home were thus situated ambiguously in the biomedical risk economy. Positioned as 'risk takers' by societal framings of homebirth as inherently risky and dangerous (Viisainen, 2000; Coxon, Sandall & Fulop, 2014), these women drew on alternative understandings of risk (as located in technology) and birthing bodies (as safe and capable) to negotiate the moral dilemmas raised by choosing to birth at home. Women choosing to birth at home and those electing to have a caesarean section did agree on one issue—that the likelihood of ending up with a caesarean section in the South African private health care system was high. However, they interpreted this differently. For women that chose caesareans, it was women's bodies that were deficient or incapable of giving birth without medical intervention.

> Hannalie: There's not a lot of women today that actually have natural deliveries, they, they try for natural (R: hmm) and then eventually it ends up being a caesarean, my gynae told me it was about three in five . . .

Rachelle: Three in five end up with a caesarean?

Hannalie: An emergency caesarean, so I dunno, I don't think they ^^make us the way they used to^^ (laughs)

In contrast, homebirthers articulated their belief in women's bodily capacity to birth without medical intervention. According to these women, it was the hospital context that was dangerous and that created a spiral of unnecessary interventions and caesarean sections. Thus, for Lizette, it was hospital birth that was risky and filled with uncertainties:

Lizette: The homebirth is so that I can make sure that nobody's going to take him away, that it will be gentle, it will be quiet, um, that I can move around and do what I need to do . . . so ja [yes] it's to try and stay out of that whole scenario [hospital] and when you go through those doors, of a hospital, your chances are, if you go through those doors you have a 65 percent chance of having a c-section, 65 percent chance.

(White, middle-class)

While homebirthers voiced belief in women's embodied capacity to give birth without medical assistance and constructed hospital birth as risky, they were none-theless deeply embedded in biomedical risk discourse. Their talk was thus haunted by anxiety-provoking and risk-infused 'what if . . . ?' questions and they reiterated that they were not opposed to technology per se but to unnecessary interventions. Importantly, the choice to birth at home was also founded on the assumption that biomedical intervention/technology and expertise was readily available and acces-sible if required. The enactment of largely middle-class notions of 'natural birth' or planned homebirth are thus founded on privileged access to resources and the ready availability of medical care and technocratic interventions on demand.

While middle-class women positioned themselves differently in relation to the possible 'risk/s to life' associated with pregnancy/birth, they were jointly located in a biomedical risk economy shaped by the commodification of biomedicine and socioeconomic privilege. This underlying privilege meant that quick access to medical care (if needed) was assumed and taken-for-granted. As explored later in this chapter, poor pregnant women in South Africa were situated very differently in relation to the biomedical risk economy. Within marginalized birth assemblages, the lives of poor women and their babies are not always highly valued. As a result, biomedical risk is enacted differently, particularly in low-tech MOUs. In these contexts, some women are subject to *invisibilization* and become 'invisible bodies' that fall outside of risk rhetoric and the medical gaze.

While normative understandings of biomedical risk shaped and framed the choices of privileged women, there were eruptions of other sources of risk in their narratives that have not been widely recognized in the literature. The corporeal vul-nerability of the laboring/birthing body to exposure, shaming, loss of control and dignity, were important risks that framed privileged women's decisions about birth.

As a result, the 'risky body' of labor/birth was not just about biomedical risk or 'risk/s to life' but was also about 'risks to self' that emerged from the corporeality of birth. Women recognized that laboring/birthing bodies were vulnerable bodies. This vulnerability was understood in different ways, depending on women's investments in particular frames of birth.

Vulnerability, risk and birthing bodies

While biomedical risk framed privileged women's talk about pregnancy and birth, there was another source of risk in their stories that centered on the fleshy vulnerability of the laboring/birthing body and attendant risks of exposure, objectification, bodily damage and mistreatment. During labor/birth, women are in unique position of bodily vulnerability—they are subject to intense pain, often overwhelming contractions and a series of psychofleshy challenges (between fragmentation and unity, self and other, inside and outside, splitting and flowing, giving and losing). Women are dependent on others for support, caregiving and physical and emotional assistance during birth. Fears and uncertainties about how the vulnerable birthing body would be treated by attendants and caregivers was thus a major concern for women. Birth choices were made *in relation* to anxieties about the heightened vulnerability and intense, often uncontrollable corporeality of the body during labor/birth. Women recognized, imagined and worried about the threats and vulnerabilities of birthing embodiment, including potential loss of bodily control, dignity and privacy, objectification and mistreatment by others, and possible damage to the sexual body. While privileged women worried about these risks and made birth choices in relation to them, it was poor women in public sector contexts that were usually the recipients of acts of mistreatment, shaming and loss of bodily dignity (see Chapter 5). As pregnant, privileged women anticipated and fantasized about birth, they negotiated, enacted and resisted sociocultural and phallocentric framings of the laboring/birthing body. Patriarchal representations of the female reproductive body and of birth as horrifying and animal-like or what Ussher (2006, p. 174) refers to as, "myths of the monstrous feminine," framed women's fears, choices, imaginings and feelings about giving birth. While women choosing elective caesareans internalized and reiterated patriarchal constructions of the birthing body as *essentially* horrifying, those that planned homebirths named medicalized birth as the problem and resisted framings of the birthing body as inherently disgusting or monstrous.

The horror of birthing bodies

Women planning elective caesareans enacted patriarchal representations of pregnancy and birth in their narratives, producing images of the laboring/birthing body as monstrous, threatening and uncontrollable (see Betterton, 2006; Ussher, 2006). Patriarchal viewpoints thus infiltrated women's imaginings of their own bodies, with affective consequences (i.e. anxiety and body–self alienation). In the talk of women choosing caesareans, the body that births was framed as horrifying and vile and associated with unacceptable risks to self and embodied dignity. Two women articulated their reasons for choosing an elective caesarean as follows:

Karin: How and why elective caesar? Frankly, I don't want my 37-year-old vagina stretched for the delivery. I don't want the risks associated with tearing, I don't want to push and sweat and moan and swear (. . .) I don't want to lie and pooh [defecate] in front of anyone—even if we manage the bowels pre-delivery.

(White, middle-class)

Taryn: I cannot imagine walking around with a day-old baby, dealing with lochia [post-birth bleeding] and urinating, all with a stitched up vagina (excuse my bluntness) (. . .) I am a very private person, I will definitely NOT like it if theatre staff stands around me while I'm lying legs in the air screaming and shouting like a mad woman.

(White, middle-class)

In these extracts, a 'nightmarish' version of birth is enacted replete with images of grotesquely stretched, torn, 'smelly' and 'stitched-up' vaginas, uncontrollable defecation, bleeding and urinating and terrifying scenes in which birthing women lie in obscene positions and are reduced to animal-like status—swearing, sweating, moaning, leaking, bursting, shouting and pushing. This is the Kristevan abject body or 'body without boundaries' par excellence, an "uncontrollable materiality" (Grosz, 1989, p. 72) that induces visceral nausea or "sickness at one's own body" (p. 75). Birth was also enacted as a degrading and humiliating event in which women became object-bodies observed by others.

Hannalie: My one friend said to me, "It's um, it's an embarrassing process to go through, to give normal birth, because you've got no control, you, you're left to these people and (*) you have to lie in an <u>obscene</u> position and it's **animal-like**."

(White, middle-class)

For women that have internalized a Western ideology of technocratic control (see Diamond, 1994) and the ideal of a self-regulated, civilized and controlled body-self, the fleshy unpredictability of birth poses significant threats to autonomy and individual control (Lupton, 1999b). Women choosing caesareans negotiated these challenges by affirming patriarchal viewpoints and disavowing aspects of their own corporeality. Internalizing denigrating ideas about birth and women's bodies, however, had unintended affective consequences that erupted in slippery ways in their talk. For example:

Hannalie: But I (*) respect the people that want to do it naturally (sighs), I just don't have, *it's not that I don't have enough faith* <u>in myself</u>, but (*) um (*) . . .

Hannalie: I think it will be a <u>nightmarish</u> experience for me, if I have to go into labor, and have to now (*) <u>rely</u> on my body ^^ to produce this baby ^^ (laughs) *Ugh*, no.

(White, middle-class)

Riddled with ambiguous meanings, Hannalie's words hint at the affective consequences of discursive enactments—in this case, a sense of body-self alienation, loss and fragmentation as she enacts her own body as unreliable, other and lacking. Patriarchal ideologies produce ontological 'truths' about women's reproductive and birthing bodies (as dirty, disgusting, animal) that circulate within birth assemblages. These ideologies enact the birthing body as a site of gendered risk, including loss of control and dignity, (sexual) objectification and exposure. As a result of their resourced positions, privileged women were able to negotiate these risks via their birth choices. At the same time, patriarchal frames continued to *affect* women's sense of self and corporeality.

While women choosing caesareans constructed birthing bodies as essentially uncontrollable and horrible and chose to opt out of the physiological birth process, homebirthers took up a different orientation to the risky corporeality of birth. For these women, the birthing body was not essentially monstrous, horrifying or a source of shame. Instead, they interpreted birth in medicalized, hospital settings as frightening, shocking and degrading (and not the fleshy birth process). For example:

Michelle: I think for me to have had it [first birth] at home took away a huge amount of anxiety and stress, um, also I think it helped me to feel like I had some form of control, and also a bit of dignity, you hear these horror stories of women exposed under these bright lights (laughs) very medicinal and impersonal (. . .) this [homebirth] is such a nice option and I think because I also had another friend who'd had a government [public sector] hospital birth and it was feet in stirrups and it was quite horrific, I mean her whole experience was shocking and that fear, I think 'oooh' (**) so it was wonderful to have another option.

(White, middle-class)

Michelle's talk is filled with references to 'anxiety,' 'fear and 'stress' as she imagines what it would be like to give birth in a (public sector) medical setting in which she would be 'exposed' and control and dignity would be lost. For her, hospital stories were "horror stories." In addition, birth in the public sector is construed as a particularly terrifying prospect and associated with extreme loss of control and dignity. Loss of dignity and bodily control thus materialized as very real risks for privileged women in relation to birth and shaped the choices they made in relation to mode and place of birth. These imagined 'risks' are suffused with sticky affective energies—fears and anxieties that have not been well recognized in the literature (or by the medical establishment) as important concerns for pregnant women. My conversations with women suggest that protecting embodied dignity and privacy are important concerns for many women in relation to birth. Jane, who gave birth at home, was clear that she was, "a private person and I don't want to be messed with" during labor. Women choosing caesareans were concerned about the very same issues. However, they chose caesarean section as the best way of trying to ensure control, dignity and bodily privacy during birth.

Through a masculinist optics

Patriarchal images of women's reproductive bodies materialized powerfully in privileged women's stories as an *outsider* perspective of birth. This outsider optics, in which birth was imagined from the perspective of an observer or audience member, was particularly prominent in the talk of women choosing caesareans. As a gendered technology of power (Chadwick & Foster, 2013), this optics emerged as a powerful frame shaping women's choices, fears and imaginings of birth. It was thus key in framing and producing the risks associated with the fleshy corporeality of birth. When speaking through this optics or patriarchal language, birthing women often became—in their discursive enactments—the *sexualized* objects of an imaginary audience. For example: "you're left to these people and (★) you have to lie in an <u>obscene</u> position and it's *animal-like*" (Hannalie). This disturbing image is suggestive of a scene in which the birthing woman is sexually objectified and horribly exposed. The entanglements between vaginal modes of birth and sex are obvious given that the vagina is an "eroticized orifice" (Grosz, 1990, p. 88). However, despite the intimate connections between sex and birth, birth is often idealized as an event (for privileged women at least) that should be pure, natural and intertwined with 'good mothering' norms (Longhurst, 2006).

Patriarchal cultures in the Global North are notoriously uncomfortable with blurred boundary lines between motherhood and sexuality, as evidenced by the widespread social anxieties surrounding public breastfeeding (Acker, 2009; Boyer, 2011). According to Longhurst (2009, p. 59), vaginal birth has the, "potential to blur the boundaries between sexual gratification and birth." As a result, birth has historically been treated as a private and intimate event, with men (including fathers) often traditionally excluded. With the shift to medicalized modes of birth in hospital settings, it is no longer true that, "giving birth is the most private of all acts" (Boden, 2015, p. 1) and most women are now required to give birth surrounded by anonymous strangers/medical professionals. The implications of this for women's sense of safety, dignity, embodied privacy and satisfaction in relation to birth has not been widely explored. Similarly, the sexual undercurrents of many obstetric practices, including the lithotomy or 'gynaecological' position and vaginal examinations, or what Bradby (1998) refers to as 'manual penetration' have not been widely investigated or debated in the literature on birth (see Kitzinger, 1992 and Bradby, 1998 as exceptions). In a rare exploration of these issues from women's perspectives, rural Bolivian women interviewed by Bradby (1998) repeatedly spoke about the sexual humiliation they experienced as a result of hospital, medicalized birth practices and described themselves as 'like a pornographic movie' for doctors *to watch*.

Women's fears and anxieties about birth often circulated with/through frightening, pornographic images of birth involving exposed genitalia and objectification. For example:

Sarah: Peter [husband] is *much* happier with a caesar, he woul(dn't), he couldn't <u>bear</u> to see me going through pain and screaming and the whole thing.

Rachelle: Ja [yes]. So this is kind of the cleaner option?

Sarah: Ja [yes], much cleaner (both laugh) it is, I mean there's also the whole issue of um, the indignity of it (. . .) just the idea of sitting there with your legs *wide* open and some midwife coming in, sticking her fingers up there every few, like every half an hour, check what's going on, *lots* of people walking in (. . .) it's something, it's a situation I can't picture myself in (R: hmm, hmm) I wouldn't want to put myself in voluntarily.

(White, middle-class)

Karin: But just to see the head on the perineum and watching these women sweating and swearing and threatening all kinds of things, it, and head here and sweat and this big, exposed area, <u>uggh</u>—no (R: okay) you know it was, I think it's also a privacy thing, you don't, I didn't really want anybody just to have a good old eyeball there (R: ja [yes]) you know it's all stretched and (*) I just didn't feel for me I wanted to be that exposed (. . .) I just emotionally couldn't cope with having to be that uncomfortable and in that position.

(White, middle-class)

In these extracts, women imagine themselves as the *objects* of an outsider optics of birth, resulting in what has been referred to as 'double consciousness' and theorized as part of a wider phenomenology of oppression (Bartky, 1990; Young, 1990a; Dolezal, 2015). Sarah and Karin thus simultaneously both imagine birth from the perspective of an objectifying external gaze and see themselves as the possible objects of this optics. Feminist literature has shown that women's sexual lives are often lived in relation to a gendered technology of doubling in which women live/experience their own bodies as potential objects subject to the judgment and appraisal of an outside other (Bartky, 1990). My conversations with privileged, pregnant women suggest that technologies of doubling in which outsider optics are internalized and used to cast the self (subject) as a potential object, also potentially apply to reproductive moments such as pregnancy and birth. Gender technologies do not only work via self-objectification but also produce feminized modes of subjectivity in which such internalized representations are 'taken up' as an integral part of the self. According to recent feminist theorizing (see Gill, 2008; Gill & Scharff, 2011), this is intimately interwoven with processes of feminine subjectification.

Birth does not exist outside of these patriarchal dynamics and the birth choices women make are intertwined with gendered technologies of power (Chadwick & Foster, 2013).

An outsider optics of birth was not confined to the talk of women choosing caesareans. Some homebirthers also drew on these images. However, an outsider optics was used to refer, not to physiological birth per se, but to medicalized birth in hospital settings. For these women, the audience point of view in relation to birth was *medicalized* and associated with the male gaze. For example:

Jane: Um, I didn't want to be at the mercy of a million doctors lying on my back with my legs up in the air, it's like—"no, way," not going there, um ja [yes], and also I don't like the idea of a male doctor looking at my bits you know (laughs).

(White, middle-class)

As expressed by Jane, in hospital she imagined that she would be, "lying on my back with my legs up in the air" with "her bits" exposed to the (male) medical gaze. Middle-class homebirthers made their decision to birth outside the hospital system in part because they wanted to ensure their own privacy and bodily dignity throughout the birth process. They did not want to become objects watched and observed by others. As Angela put it: "I want people there as support as opposed to spectators, I really don't want people sitting there watching me." The risk of being objectified, shamed and observed as a spectacle during labor/birth were therefore significant concerns. Decisions about how/where to give birth were made in relation to these fears and anxieties. Most middle-class women planning homebirths were also concerned with the risks of *losing control* in medicalized, hospital settings. For example, Jane was clear in saying she chose to birth at home because, "I wanted control" and according to Daniella she was, "really scared of doctors taking away your power (. . .) or making you feel like out-of-control." It must be noted that 'homebirthers' are not a homogenous group all defined by white privilege and middle-class status. During the research process, I talked to two black, low-income women who had planned homebirths with private midwives. Their homebirth stories were not about negotiating the corporeal risky body that births or preventing loss of control—as I will show in the next section, planned homebirth was sometimes about other risks, centering significantly around lack of care in the public health care system. It is thus important that we remain cautious about treating public and private as fixed, homogenous categories that map seamlessly onto race, privilege and socioeconomics.

Privileged South African women were thus embedded in risk economies shaped by high-tech obstetrics, patriarchal ideologies and racialized socioeconomics. Birth in the private sector was shaped powerfully by normative discourses of biomedical risk, which operated within a particular privatized bioeconomy structured by wealth, privilege and the commodification of health services, technology and expertise. Within this biomedical risk economy, most pregnancies and births are highly monitored and hypervisible, subject to repeated and intensive surveillance and testing, and shaped by discourses of technoscience, medical expertise, individual responsibilization and the inherent dangers of physiological birth. At the same time, there were also *other* sources of risk circulating within privileged risk economies. Women recognized the corporeal vulnerability of labor/birth and were worried about risks of exposure, loss of dignity, mistreatment and objectification. Problematically, patriarchal 'truths' about the ontology of birthing bodies (i.e. as essentially horrifying, threatening and shameful) framed these corporeal risks, often in alienating ways. Patriarchal frames materialized as an 'outside optics' of labor/birth in which women imagined themselves as the potential objects of the abjecting gaze, resulting in the vertigo of double consciousness. Privileged women, however, negotiated these risk economies in different ways, some internalized phallocentric images and abjected aspects of their own corporeality, choosing caesarean section as a means of negating the bodily risks of birth, while others identified medicalization and hospital birth as the source of corporeal risks during birth and gave birth at home.

The risk/s of lack of care

While privileged women were concerned with the risk of 'losing control' and made birth choices accordingly, worries about 'control' did not appear in the stories of low-income women. This confirms previous findings that the concept of 'control' lacks salience for women of marginalized sociomaterial locations (Nelson, 1983; Lazarus, 1997; Zadoroznyj, 1999). Maintaining self-control over the body that births was not a key concern in the stories of low-income women. For these women, entangled within a different set of risk politics, a key concern in relation to birth was not loss of control but lack of *care*.

'Care' had multiple meanings in women's stories and referred both to adequate medical attention and monitoring and humane, supportive treatment by caregivers. While birth choices were limited for these women, with most having little option other than to utilize public maternity services, I did talk to two low-income, black women who were slightly more resourced (but still did not have private medical aid) who actively sought out private midwifery care after unpleasant experiences in the public sector. I interviewed Tasneem, a Muslim woman living in a house situated in a more upmarket suburb of the Cape Flats, in the late stages of her second pregnancy. We talked about her decision to have her baby at home with a private midwife and her previous experience of giving birth in a local MOU.

Tasneem: We had no medical aid and things like that, so um (. . .) at that point in time, so when I, um, so the only way to go was provincially [public sector], okay, and there's this day clinic that we had to attend, and then the local MOU in X, that was the only choice that we had, um, so far it went well, but the **actual** birth it was quite traumatic, because um, being the first time, I was about 20 years old, you know, the care that was given wasn't what I expected.

Tasneem repeatedly described her first birth experience at the public sector MOU as, "very much traumatic," because she was afforded no *sense of care* from the nurses on duty. Instead of comforting her and making her feel at ease during her first birth, the nurses were impatient, negative and unhelpful. As a result, they said things like, "Oh, you're not supposed to be here" even when it turned out that she was in advanced labor (eight centimeters dilated) and "Come on woman you must push the baby's head." According to Tasneem, she was lucky that she had her mother-in-law with her, "as a comforter, wiping me off with the sweat and things like that." As a first time mother, she did not, "know **what** to do" or "**how** to push" and was filled with uncertainty and anxiety. Tasneem was also not afforded any dignity or respect as a woman who had just given birth and was, "left all alone" after delivery and told, "here's a bucket and you clean yourself."

As a result of her traumatic first birth, Tasneem explored other options when she fell pregnant with her second baby. A friend recommended that she consult Sharon, a private midwife. At this stage, Tasneem was clear that the thought of having a homebirth, "never crossed my mind" and that she "just wanted **care**." Unlike the privileged women in the study who usually turned to homebirth as a search for control and a desire to, "feel that sense of ownership" (Erin) in relation to birth, Tasneem was motivated by a need to avoid the risks of trauma and lack of care and secure engaged and supportive care during labor/birth.

> *Tasneem:* I just wanted **care** you know cause I didn't want to go through that trauma [of first birth] you know (. . .) and then we hooked up with Sharon [private midwife] (. . .) I was very much impressed with the whole, you know, this whole care that she gave us, to me, it was "I'm the most important thing here" cause I'm carrying something **special** here, you know, that was, that just made, it was very overwhelming, just receiving this care, not having anything the first time around.

Towards the end of her pregnancy, Tasneem had to decide whether to give birth in the only local public hospital that was "midwife-friendly" (i.e. allowed the use of a private midwife) or to give birth at home attended by midwife Sharon. This decision was made by weighing up biomedical risk factors against the 'risks to self' of giving birth in a public hospital (i.e. trauma and lack of supportive care). While drawing on biomedical risk discourse to frame her view that homebirth was safe: "everything was fine, blood levels were fine, sugar was fine so it was less likely for complications," she reiterates that, "I wanted Sharon to deliver my baby." Ultimately, care was favored over the biomedical safety promised by hospital and biomedical technology.

> *Tasneem:* . . . maybe if you're at the hospital um you'd feel more safer but the care you got, there wasn't that care, here you're at home and you've got this care so it was more reassuring, you know, you felt more comfortable.

Tasneem's narrative shows that 'homebirth' is not one thing. Tasneem's home-birth was framed in relation to the importance of guaranteeing care and support during labor/birth. Utilizing a private midwife became a way of avoiding the risks to self rampant in the public sector, including the possibility of more 'trauma,' mistreatment and lack of care. While giving birth in a private hospital was not an option for Tasneem (she did not have private medical aid or sufficient financial resources), a planned homebirth offered an intermediate path to better levels of care. Tasneem's case shows that planned homebirth is not a mode of birth relevant only to middle-class, privileged women seeking a 'natural birth' but that home-birth with a private midwife can be a route towards dignity, care and support for some marginalized women.

'Risk politics' in marginalized birth assemblages

It's life and death also—you or the child.

(Jasmine, black, very poor)

Given rampant socioeconomic inequality rooted in historical legacies of colonization and apartheid, the statistical risks of death during pregnancy, birth and the early post-partum are substantially higher for low-income South African women in the public sector than they are for women receiving care in the private sector. In South Africa, disparities in maternal mortality rates for private and public sectors mirror global disjunctures in maternal deaths between North/South rooted in racial and socioeco-nomic equalities. These disparities are evidence of the life-and-death consequences of embodied inequalities (Spangler, 2011). In South Africa, women giving birth in public sector settings are more than seven times more likely to die during birth than women accessing private health care services (see Bateman, 2014). Driven by bioeconomics, profit and commodification, risk technologies do not always operate according to the logic of need. As a result, biomedical technologies often intensify where they are least needed and are missing in contexts where they are most needed (Johnson, 2016). This is true both in South Africa and on a global scale.

Framing 'risk politics' in relation to pregnancy and birth are thus large-scale material configurations of power, exclusion, resources, infrastructure, capitali-zation and compounding historical legacies involving racialized patriarchy and colonization. These sociomaterial relations result in the production of different risk economies for middle-class women in private health care settings and low-income women in the public sector. The most marginalized of South African women have little choice but to birth in public sector conditions. As noted earlier however, 'pri-vate' and 'public' are not neat, homogenous and fixed categories that always map seamlessly onto race (i.e. some low-income white women give birth in the public sector and there are increasing numbers of middle-class black women utilizing pri-vate health care). Furthermore, it must be noted that the public and private sectors are comprised of multiple contexts and terrains—for example, the public sector is a mix of highly medicalized tertiary-level hospitals, intermediate district hospitals and low-technology MOUs run predominantly by nurse-midwives. The private maternity sector is generally highly medicalized and technocratic. However, some private hospitals allow the use of private midwives and doulas while others do not. Furthermore, women giving birth at home with private midwives are also considered broadly part of the private (paying) health care system.

The particular sociopolitical geographies in which birth takes place have material consequences for the emergence of different risk economies. In tertiary level public hospitals, low-income women are subject to high levels of technocratic medicalization during labor and treated via narrow definitions of biomedical risk. In public sector MOUs however, the biomedical risk economy is structured very differently and in some settings is marked by the absence of technological monitoring and machinery, indifferent care and a lack of surveillance. In these contexts, women's laboring bodies are often rendered invisible and fall outside of biomedical optics. There are thus multiple 'risk economies' that materialize across different public health settings. At the same time, differences exist in the broad ways in which pregnant and laboring bodies are inscribed by the practices, norms and discourses of biomedical risk across private and public sector divides. While women utilizing the private medical sector are usually highly monitored throughout their pregnancies, poor pregnant women are generally not subject to the same degree of high-tech monitoring and risk management. Most low-income women that I spoke to had only one ultrasound (and some women had none) during their pregnancies, while middle-class women attended by private medical specialists easily had more than six sonograms as well as additional and more advanced 3D and 4D ultrasounds at specialized foetal assessment centers. In the public sector, ultrasounds are used in a strictly routine and diagnostic fashion (women are not routinely even given an ultrasound photograph), unlike in the private sector where ultrasounds function as key social moments in the narrative of pregnancy and are intertwined with neoliberal modes of (pregnancy, birth, mothering) consumption (see Taylor, 2000; Taylor, Layne & Wozniak, 2004). The degree to which biomedical risk technologies are entangled with profit, modes of consumption and neoliberal capitalism needs greater acknowledgment and exploration. What has been predominantly highlighted in the literature thus far is not the exclusionary dimensions of biomedicalization and technocratic risk technologies but the "postmodern intertwining" of health care and middle-class, neoliberal consumerism (often in contexts of the Global North) where individuals are provided with enabling "techniques for exploring new horizons of self-development and self-actualization" (Thompson, 2003, p. 83). This was certainly applicable to the privileged women interviewed, where pregnancy and birth often became an identity-making process in which a range of technologies and practices (3D sonograms, acupuncture, pregnancy yoga, amniocentesis, hypno-birthing) were used as 'technologies of the self' to craft selves and identities (Foucault, 1997).

Sociomaterially marginalized women were largely excluded from discourses of neoliberal 'choice' and enactments of mothering identities via modes of consumption because of their socioeconomic situations. Socioeconomics shape risk politics, resulting in the emergence of different risk economies for privileged, resourced women and low-income women. As a result of socioeconomics, the commodification of biomedical technology and expertise and legacies of structural inequality, women in public sector contexts lacked the array of birth choices available to middle-class women. As a result, they could not (usually) seek extra medical testing or decide to have an elective caesarean section. Driven by a different set of sociomaterial forces, 'risk' was articulated and enacted differently. While fears concerning 'risks to life' continued to frame women's birth experiences in public sector assemblages, there were other 'risks to self' circulating in relation to birth that were at times more significant. These 'risks' included: the risk/s of poverty, lack of care and mistreatment (explored fully in Chapter 5).

Poverty and its risks

> I don't have <u>anything</u>, anything.
>
> *(Jasmine, black, very poor)*

While Tasneem (see pages 88-90) was able to find a way of exiting the public health care system in her second pregnancy, most low-income women did not have such options. The high levels of poverty that most low-income women in this study experienced meant that the only 'choice' was birth in the public sector or birth at home with no health care provider. Jasmine, who was living in conditions of abject poverty with three children (in a back room) with virtually no furniture, electricity or income, decided on the latter. According to Jasmine, she did not attend the local MOU for antenatal care or 'book-in' for the birth because of her anxiety about what the local nurse-midwives would say about her poverty and how she would be treated as a result of it.

> *Jasmine:* No, I wasn't *there* [at MOU], the reason why is, um, private problems, I was shy, I was afraid also of what people were gonna say, I told [counsellor] that was my main reason also that I didn't go book also *and* I didn't have kimbies [disposable nappies], I didn't have baby clothes, see I was well off before—what are people gonna say if *I* uh (*) gonna *give birth* like that (R: hmm).
>
> *(Black, very poor)*

Jasmine did not attend antenatal services and made no plans to register or 'book in' for the birth of her baby because of a deep sense of shame about her poverty, multiparity (this was her third baby) and lack of baby goods (nappies and clothes). She was anxious about what would be said about her and wanted to avoid being shamed, gossiped about and censured. As a result, she gave birth at home with no health care provider present to assist with the delivery. In addition to being scared about how she would be judged and humiliated for her poverty at the public sector MOU, Jasmine was also scared of being mistreated. She talked about being humiliated by nurses during her previous birth experiences.

Jasmine: There are three sisters [nurses] that I'm very scared of, they're RUDE.
Rachelle: At the clinic?
Jasmine: Yes, they're RUDE, they will just tell you, they will say, "No, you did that [sex] *lekker* [lustfully]"—that kind of stuff, they will, because I remember from, with X [previous baby] I was supposed to walk up and down, up and down, up and down and they were sitting in a room, they were sitting in a room and when you say the pain is coming or you go to the bed, they will **shout** at you, <u>ugly</u> remarks, they will, they will gi(ve), that, that was also one of my reasons because they're gonna treat me like that, because I was scared, I've got three children also, now they're gonna say, they're RUDE man.

(Black, very poor)

Jasmine thus opted to take the risk of birthing at home with no caregiver or birth attendant rather than face potential humiliation, shaming and mistreatment at the local health-services. Even when she was in labor and neighbors were trying to encourage her to go to the local clinic, Jasmine continued to steadfastly refuse.

Jasmine: . . . the neighbors, the neighbors are very supportive, the neighbors <u>came</u> and I was sitting there, "***Come, come*** to the doctor" but they, they do(n't) they don't **<u>understand</u>**—the pain also but the other thing was that I don't want to go cause then ↑*they're gonna skel* [**shout at**] *me out also*↑ (R: okay)

Jasmine knew that she had taken a risk by not attending antenatal care and giving birth at home with no caregiver; she noted, "I must take full responsibility." However, later in the interview she expressed delight that the birth had taken place successfully at home and that she had managed to avoid the problems, difficulties and 'risks to self' of giving birth in the local public-sector maternity clinic.

Jasmine: ^^I'm very glad^^ (both laugh) ^^I'M VERY GLAD IT HAPPENED HERE^^ I'm very glad and it was quick also but I think #
Rachelle: Did you feel like you had a lot of support [from neighbors]?
Jasmine: I had a lot of support, a lot of support yes and I went to go thank everyone, it was a nice experience.
Rachelle: So it was actually better for you than the other ones that you had at the clinic?
Jasmine: Yes, it's much better, it's much better
Rachelle: Why?

Jasmine: My own space, yes, my own space and also, you would have had the pain there also—the, the sisters they would've walked up and down the whole time, they will <u>ignore</u> you because I had that experience before also with X and Y also, they will ignore you, it's almost like—"You don't talk the truth, you don't know when the baby is gonna come" that kind of stuff, yes, but it was good, it was good yes, but it's life and death also—you or the child . . .

Jasmine's sense of happiness and satisfaction with her homebirth was tempered by the recognition of the 'risk/s to life' that she had taken by forgoing any kind of medical assistance during pregnancy/birth. As she put it, "it was good yes, but it's life and death also—you or the child." Jasmine believed that her poverty and multiparity put her at heightened risk for public shaming and mistreatment by nurses at the local MOU. She was thus willing to face 'life-and-death' risks rather than suffer "the pain there" of being ignored, humiliated and treated rudely. Jasmine was not the only poor woman to emphasize the risks of poverty *over* biomedical risks in relation to birth. Consider the following exchange:

Rachelle: And were you scared about the birth before the time?
Carmen: Ask X [community counsellor], I told her I was SCARED (laughs) very, very scared, cause I wasn't <u>prepared</u> (*) but then #
Rachelle: So how, what do you mean by not prepared?
Carmen: Like with, with <u>stuff</u> for him, I was (. . .) I <u>need</u> stuff, there was stuff that I needed so I was a bit worried . . .

As a middle-class interviewer steeped in normative understandings of fear and risk as predominantly about biomedical risk and complications, I had difficulty in hearing what Carmen was trying to tell me about her distinctive fears as a poor pregnant woman. Rather than being scared about the possibilities of biomedical risk, she was worried about not having enough supplies and baby goods. Later in the interview I again struggled to hear her (from my middle-class positioning).

Rachelle: Okay, so there were quite a lot of complications—was that part of why you were scared?
Carmen: Mhmmm (*)↑**I was actually scared**↑ cause I didn't have enough stuff, so there were complications but that wasn't my problem, my problem was I didn't have enough stuff for him (*) I was a bit scared (R: okay)

While I kept on referring to complications and biomedical risks, Carmen kept coming back to the very material issue of not having sufficient baby supplies. For her this was a serious concern because it would mark her out as 'poor' and as potentially a 'bad mother' (who was not sufficiently 'prepared') in the local clinic. Pregnant women are instructed to bring a certain amount of baby supplies (disposable nappies, soap, baby clothes, baby toiletries) with them to the MOU when they give birth. Not being able to meet these requirements and bring sufficient supplies puts poor women at risk for stigmatization, shaming and mistreatment. For low-income women in the public sector, 'risks' in relation to birth were not only about 'risks to life' in the form of possible biomedical complications and death. Risk was a broader concept that encompassed a set of possible 'risks to self' and dignity in public sector contexts. Being singled out as 'poor' and possibly a 'bad mother' as a result of having insufficient baby goods, being shamed, mistreated and ignored were material and affective risks to self that low-income women had to negotiate during birth in public sector birth assemblages. In Jasmine's case, she was prepared to risk her life and that of her child by giving birth at home without a birth attendant so that she could avoid the risk of a loss of dignity and public humiliation in the MOU. While 'risks to life' frame the birth event for both middle-class and low-income women, poverty brings particular 'risks to self' that only low-income women had to negotiate.

Becoming invisible: the politics of erasure

^^They forgot about me, they didn't even know I was *there*^^

(Wendy, black, low-income)

It is often assumed that biomedicalization operates via heightened surveillance, monitoring and a raft of risk technologies in relation to birth. As a result, hospitals are typically regarded as panoptical settings in which laboring bodies become subject to hypervisibility (Arney, 1982; Simonds, 2002). According to Arney (1982, p. 150), monitoring has become, "the new order of obstetrical power." In Arney's (1982) Foucauldian analysis of the history of obstetrics, he argues that obstetrics has shifted from being an oppressive and 'top-down' form of power to being characterized by the all-seeing, "normalizing gaze" (p. 88) of panopticism. While the power and intensity of the biomedical gaze is substantial in private sector obstetric contexts in South Africa, the medical gaze is uneven in the public sector.

Shifts in South African forms of governance and State power from apartheid to democracy has left indelible traces on the public health care system. As a result of legacies of inequality, racial oppression and lack of infrastructure and resources, the medical gaze often falters in the public sector, with some patients becoming 'invisible' (Gibson, 2004). While the geography of public hospital wards and clinics in South Africa are still spatially designed and organized to maximize patient visibility and surveillance, in reality patients are sometimes, "lost in transit while in foyers, in waiting-rooms, and between wards" (Gibson, 2004, p. 2017). Kruger and Schoombie (2010, p. 97) have argued that despite the fundamental principles of biomedicalization or "order, surveillance, intervention, risk-aversion" being apparent in public sector obstetric settings, the medical gaze is often uneven, patchy and sometimes absent. According to Foucault, the medical gaze functions as a technology of power that 'disciplines' the body of the patient and makes it the object of biomedical categorization and normalizing techniques (Foucault, 1980). Kruger and Schoombie (2010) however argue that chaos and disorganization are often the order of the day in public sector obstetric settings and the "ideals of the medicalised discourse" (p. 97) are rarely successfully implemented. These 'gaps in the gaze' (Gibson, 2004) are, in my view, important *sites of differings* where biomedicalization intra-acts with other sociomaterialities to produce different articulations of biomedical power.

'Risk' materializes differently according to context, and biomedical power is enacted via differing relations of visibility/invisibility depending on wider material, socioeconomic and relational dynamics. As noted by Casper and Moore (2009, p. 9): "because society is stratified along lines of gender, race, class, sexuality, age, disability status, citizenship, geography, and other cleavages, some bodies are public and visually dissected while others are vulnerable to erasure and marginalization."

The optics of biomedical power thus involve not only the hypervisibility and surveillance of bodies but also marginalizing modes of erasure, disappearance, invisibility and forgetting. Biomedical power is diffractively enacted within birth assemblages and processes of visibility/invisibility *both* function as techniques of power. According to Gordon (1996), the visible and the invisible need to be recognized as intimately interconnected. Pregnancy and birth are potentially subject to complex forms of both surveillance, panoptical monitoring and hypervisibility and processes of erasure and invisibility. For example, subjecting the interior of the pregnant body to the clinical gaze via ultrasound technologies paradoxically makes the pregnant body and the unborn fetus 'hypervisible' and yet, simultaneously, often renders the personhood and subjectivity of the pregnant woman invisible (Taylor, 2008; Macleod & Howell, 2015). Medical technologies thus work ambiguously to both make visible and erase or mute, often at the same time.

Biomedical techniques and the clinical gaze are also sometimes withheld or unavailable and some bodies are treated as if they were disposable and left to die (see Gibson, 2004). While linked to structural inequalities, health system inadequaces and lack of resources, at the same time, processes of invisibilization in the South African public health care system are also wider operations of societal power. Sociopolitical relations frame some lives (white, able-bodied, middle-class, Christian, heterosexual) as valuable and others (black, poor, queer) as disposable (Butler, 2016). Processes whereby black and poor laboring bodies are rendered invisible and left to fall outside of normative modes of biomedical risk management (in some public sector contexts) speak to wider forms of societal power in which some lives are valued (and must be protected) and others are not. Both the panoptical gaze and the absence or withholding of the gaze thus function as potential technologies of power and are embedded in sociomaterial relations of oppression, privilege and marginalization.

In the public sector, women were subject to different kinds of risk economies. Close analysis of birth stories thus found that there is no generic and undifferentiated 'public sector' in South Africa, nor is there any homogenous form of biomedical power. Some women in the public sector were subject to high-tech monitoring and risk management while others were not. Women giving birth in public tertiary-level hospitals were thus often marked as 'high risk' and subject to substantial degrees of biomedical surveillance, monitoring and technocratic interventions. Hierarchies between patients and experts and the valorization of technology, machines and biomedical expertise were clearly delineated. The authoritative status of medical staff was enacted via technocratic interventions and standard use of bureaucratic and objectifying techniques and hierarchical relations. Women were often more satisfied with their births (although there were exceptions) in these settings and felt more 'cared for' because they were monitored and subject to the medical gaze.

Tracy: They [nurses in public hospital setting] did proper checks on me (★) and they cleaned me and things like that and I was treated much better there and I got my antibiotics and things.

> *(Black, low-income, MOU labor transferred to public hospital)*

Rachelle: So the nurses—the treatment was good at the hospital?
Vanessa: Very good yes because the room where I lay, they, the sisters that were on duty, they come <u>in the morning</u>, the evening and uuh give you *pills* and everyone that needs pills, asks for pills and so . . .

> *(Black, low-income, MOU labor transferred to public hospital)*

Biomedical modes of birth characterized by regular medical attention were thus often well-received. Several women experienced pills, examinations, checks, machines and information as comforting. Women also spoke about actively desiring monitoring and the biomedical gaze, which for many was equivalent to 'care.' As argued by Pylypa (1998), biopower operates centrally through the production of desire in the individual to engage in modes of discipline and normalization. Furthermore, following Foucault (1980, p. 59), it is important to emphasize the point that power, "produces effects at the level of desire." While medicalization was well received by some, other women were frustrated by the ways in which machines constrained their freedom and embodied agency during labor.

Madiha: **I ask, I ask**, I ask them—can't they just make this thing [electronic foetal monitor] *looser* because the pain comes at the back and <u>that thing</u> is ↑*tight, tight, tight*↑ and then they said, "No, that thing is because the baby's heart," to monitor the baby's heart and that (. . .) I couldn't even walk <u>because</u> {*the drips are all here in my hands*} (. . .) now you can't lie on your back, you have to lie on your side the whole time so that <u>that thing</u> can (★) monitor the baby.

> *(Black, low-income, public hospital birth)*

Celeste: When they give you pains [induction] you must just lay on one side, the, the heartbeat, the one that listens to the baby's heartbeat, <u>so you must just lay for 16 hours</u>, you must just lay on one side (. . .) it's terrible to lay 16 hours just on one side and you can't even **move** but that's, if they give you pains that's what you deal with.

(Black, low-income, public hospital birth)

While it has been argued that the critique of medicalization during birth only resonates with "privileged populations" (Johnson, 2016, p. 47), the stories of low-income women show a more nuanced reality in which medicalization is both desired, sometimes withheld and also experienced by some women as oppressive.

While many women actively desired modes of medicalization to make them feel safe, these needs and desires often went unmet in MOU settings. In clinic settings women are assumed to be 'low-risk' and routinely left to labor alone without medical interventions or drugs; they often had what in middle-class vocabularies would constitute undisrupted, 'natural' births. However, in contexts where care and monitoring were absent, these births were not regarded by women as 'empowering.' Often they were left distressed by a lack of medical monitoring and assistance. With risk management, surveillance and assessments often absent, women described a process of *becoming invisible* in which they were disregarded, lost and forgotten.

Wendy: And then I, I went to the sister to ask her how far I was and she said she had completely forgotten about me ^^they forgot about me, they didn't even know I was *there*^^ ja [yes] and then she said um, "I must go on waiting, she will be with me soon" and then I **waited** and (⋆) *um* (⋆⋆) um then walked up and down (⋆) some of the sisters is *just busy* with ↑*other things*↑

Rachelle: What sort of things?

Wendy: ^^They don't worry about us^^, *uuh*, like ⋆on the computer⋆ playing games *and so* (⋆) uh, th(at), that solitaire games (⋆) ja [yes] ^^on the computer^^ (giggles) (R laughs) they don't worry about us (⋆) I, I, I don't think it's, it's not actually right.

In this snippet, Wendy is 'forgotten' by the nurses who she says, "didn't even know I was there." In MOU contexts, biomedical risk management and the medical gaze often seemed to evaporate as laboring bodies were left unmonitored. According to Rosetta, "I basically gave birth alone." Women described being left alone for hours, sometimes shouting or screaming for help and receiving no response. Wendy thus described the scenario at the MOU as one in which laboring women, "walked around ^^some **screamed**, some lay on the bed, some went to call the nurses but nobody came^^ *to help*." Nurses were depicted as busy elsewhere, "doing their own thing" (Vanessa). Several women also reported that they were instructed by nurses to only call for assistance when delivery was imminent. As a result, some women were at risk of delivering their babies alone and unattended.

Sanele: They didn't check, they say (★) if *you* feel like the baby's coming you must go and (★★) you must go to the bed

Rachelle: And then?

Sanele: Then you must call for them (. . .) so I go *there*, I open the door and I say "Nurse, I feel like the head is coming out."

(MOU birth)

Madiha: . . . then I felt the baby's head is going to come out, then I wanted to walk there [to nurses] but then I saw that I can't {*can't walk*}, then I screamed "*Sister*, the baby is coming now!" then she said, "No, go and lie on the bed man, the baby isn't coming now" and then (★) then I said to the other girl [patient], "Go and tell the sister he baby is coming now" because the head had already come out, then she went to tell and then they came running (★) and then they got their things together.

(Black, low-income, MOU birth)

Giving birth in a South African MOU is thus no guarantee of receiving bio-medical assistance or even having a skilled birth attendant present during delivery. Such blatant neglect and disregard leaves women feeling abandoned, unworthy and unsafe. It is also potentially dangerous and irresponsible as some women give birth with little medical assistance—i.e. as in Madiha's case where, "the head had already come out" before medical personnel arrived to help. In MOU contexts, the birth stories of poor women were pervaded by a sense of institutional disregard for their welfare communicated to them by systemic practices of neglect, lack of care and invisibilization. They became 'invisible bodies' that did not matter. In these settings, standard biomedical protocols of risk management, surveillance and monitoring were often absent and laboring women were left wandering around corridors feeling lost and/or endlessly waiting for some kind of medical assessment. Not subject to regular monitoring or the biomedical gaze, women described nurses as negligent and uncaring. Disinterest in patients and lack of 'care' (monitoring) emerged in women's stories as normative in MOU settings. This invisibilization of laboring women also had *affective consequences*, making them feel insignificant, invisible and unworthy of biomedical attention. It also reiterated broader social relations of power according to which the lives/bodies of poor, black pregnant women are regarded as disposable.

Summary

This chapter explored 'risk politics' as enacted in women's birth stories. 'Risk' in relation to birth was shown to be heterogeneous and diffractive, with enactments of risk differing according to socioeconomic positions. While 'risk' in relation to birth is often assumed to narrowly mean 'biomedical risk,' this chapter showed that women negotiate multiple risks in relation to birth, depending on their locations. While the chapter troubled the notion that 'public' and 'private' health care sectors were fixed, stable and homogenous spaces, there were nonetheless important differences in the structuring of risk politics across public–private divides. Women situated in the private sector were embedded in a risk economy dominated by high-tech obstetrics, surveillance medicine and the valorization of biomedical expertise. Structured by socioeconomic principles of commodification, privatization and capitalization, women's pregnant and birthing bodies were subject to hypervisibility via frequent monitoring and obstetric testing. In this risk economy, 'risks to life' were central and biomedical technologies and expertise were seen as guardians of life. Biomedical risk economies were vitalized by ontological framings of the body that births as essentially risky, unpredictable and prone to dysfunction. Some women embraced medicalization and biomedical risk politics, choosing caesarean sections for reasons of safety and predictability. Others resisted narrow framings of biomedical risk and the birthing body as a source of risk and dysfunction. Women planning homebirths were shown to be ambiguously positioned in relation to biomedical risk discourse and practices, both rejecting and reiterating biomedical risk vocabularies. Enactments of biomedical risk were therefore not homogenous in privileged, private sector birth assemblages. At the same time, women embedded in resourced and privileged locations took the ready availability of medical services and obstetric interventions for granted. The decision to birth at home was thus premised on easy access to biomedical technologies if/when needed.

While biomedical risk served as an overarching frame vitalizing the everyday politics of birth, the chapter argued that there were also *other* sources of risk that framed and shaped women's birth choices and experiences. In the case of privileged women, the 'risky body' of birth was not just biomedically risky; women also articulated their fears and concerns about the 'risks to self' posed by the vulnerable corporeality of the body that births. The embodied risks of birth included: loss of control, exposure, objectification and threats to dignity, privacy and bodily integrity. Some women spoke in/through phallocentric languages of birth, framing the leaking, bursting, spilling, pulsating and fragmenting laboring/birthing body as *essentially* monstrous, repugnant and horrifying. As a result, elective caesareans were seen by some as a mode of escape from the monstrous corporeality of labor/birth and the threats it posed to selfhood, agency, order and containability. Patriarchal ideologies of birth, reproduction and women's bodies were vitalized and enacted via an outsider optics in which women imagined themselves through the objectifying and abjecting masculinist gaze. While some women internalized this gaze and abjected aspects of their own corporeality, others resisted and framed it as a medicalized, male-centered and distorting optics. Women planning homebirths thus framed the corporeal risks of labor/birth (exposure, shaming, loss of dignity) as products of medicalized, hospital birth rather than inherent to women's bodies. Private sector risk economies were thus shown to be highly technocratic, racialized and patriarchal socioeconomies, driven by biomedical risk discourse. Laboring/birthing bodies materialized as essentially risky, monstrous and unpredictable through the ontological frames of patriarchal biomedicine. While 'risks to life' are central to biomedical risk economies, women also worried about the 'risks to self' vitalized in/through ontological framings of the birthing body as abject, uncontainable and threatening.

Risk politics was enacted differently in the birth stories of low-income women. For many of these women, the greatest threat/s in relation to birth were not loss of control or sexualized objectification but poverty and lack of care and medical assistance. For some women, poverty was constructed as a major source of risk. Being visibly marked as 'poor' (often via lack of baby supplies) meant that women's moral identities as 'good mothers' were put into question. Furthermore, being marked as 'poor' also resulted in stigmatization and the intensification of possible mistreatments in public sector services (particularly MOUs). Some women regarded the risk/s of being outed as poor as more frightening than the possibility of biomedical complications/risks. The 'public sector' was not homogenous but comprised of different risk economies. In public hospitals, usually reserved for women deemed to be 'high risk,' sociomaterial and technocratic practices structured by the logic/ parameters of biomedical risk were dominant. In these settings women were often subject to high levels of medicalization (electronic foetal monitors, intravenous drips, pharmacologic and surgical interventions). Many low-income women welcomed medicalized forms of birth and practices of risk management and monitoring, measurements, drugs and assessments were often regarded as evidence of 'care.' Others were, however, frustrated by the oppressive constraints of obstetric technologies. In MOU settings, biomedical risk protocols materialized unevenly. Standard operations of biomedical power via high levels of monitoring, physical examination and stringent forms of risk management were often absent in these contexts as women narrated being left alone, 'forgotten' and unmonitored. I argue that biomedical risk economies materialized via a politics of both hypervisibility and invisibility in different contexts. In MOU settings, low-income women were often subject to processes of *invisibilization*, which marked them as bodies/lives that did not matter and as unworthy of medical care and assessment. Larger sociomaterial and socioeconomic power relations in South Africa that inscribe some bodies as worthy of protection, risk management and respect and other bodies as disposable, unrecognized, unworthy and invisible, circulate within birth assemblages. Furthermore, like the panoptical gaze, invisibilization functions as a technology of biomedical power that reiterates power hierarchies and disciplines laboring/ birthing bodies.

5
VIOLATED BODIES

Birth violence has been reported since the 1950s (Goer, 2010), with Euro-American feminists at the forefront of activism, research and debate in this area (Rich, 1986; Martin, 1987; Kitzinger, 1992). However, it is only since the 2000s that birth violence has been recognized as a global health problem (D'Oliveira, Diniz & Schraibe, 2002). More recently, several position statements have called for global attention and accelerated efforts to address this violence (Freedman & Kruk, 2014; WHO, 2014; Jewkes & Penn-Kekana, 2015). Contestations and ontological politics, however, abound in debates about birth violence. Deciding what to call this violence has been a problem, with competing terms (i.e. childbirth abuse, mistreatment, traumatic birth, disrespectful care and obstetric violence) used by scholars/ activists operating in different contexts, disciplines and political fields. The terms and frames used to think about birth violence are thus sticky with conceptual and contextual politics that mirror the broader politics of birth (see Chapter 2). Work on birth violence is situated complexly between disciplines, geopolitical zones (North/South) and activisms. Since the 2000s, most research on birth violence has been dominated by public health and biomedical approaches and has not been overtly political. There has thus been a tendency to conceptualize birth violence as a narrow interpersonal affair, frame it within vocabularies of 'trauma' (Mozingo et al., 2002; Moyzakitis, 2004; Baker, Choi & Henshaw, 2005; Thomson & Downe, 2008; Elmir et al., 2010) or see it as indicative of the failure of evidence-based medicine or problems in generic 'health systems' (Rattner et al., 2007; Van den Broek & Graham, 2009; Mathai, 2011; Vogel et al., 2016).

However, the rise of the concept of 'obstetric violence' in contexts of the Global South has disrupted depoliticized readings of birth violence. Emerging as a legal term in Latin and Central America over the last decade, obstetric violence criminalizes acts of abuse and inhumane care during birth in certain countries (currently Venezuela, Argentina and Mexico). Unlike terms such as mistreatment, abuse, trauma and disrespectful care, obstetric violence is firmly rooted in birth activist movements to humanize birth in Latin America. As a result, the term is overtly political and provocative and linked to efforts to critique social relations of marginalization embedded in gender, class and race oppressions (Dixon, 2015; Smith-Oka, 2015). According to Dixon (2015, p. 450), references to obstetric violence are, "unexpected, jarring and provocative" and deliberately used by activists to challenge abusive practices that have often been hidden or normalized during birth. As a result, the term is controversial and has been received with hostility by medical professionals in Latin America (Dixon, 2015). Importantly, the concept of obstetric violence is embedded in legal vocabularies that name it as a form of gender violence. Thus far, few studies in Northern settings have utilized the term 'obstetric violence.' However, the term is becoming a traveling concept and is increasingly being taken up in a range of settings (see Pickles, 2015; Diaz-Tello, 2016; Shabot, 2016; Chadwick, 2017b). Moreover, since 2014, five obstetric violence observatories (civil rights groups) have been founded in diverse geopolitical settings including Chile, France, Argentina, Columbia and Spain (Sadler et al., 2016).

The increasing circulatory power of the term obstetric violence across transnational boundaries has meant an increasing recognition of intersecting power relations in articulations of birth violence. While earlier efforts to define birth abuse referred only to four forms of direct violence, namely: physical abuse, verbal abuse, sexual abuse and neglect (see D'Oliveira, Diniz & Schraibe, 2002), recent definitions have shifted towards an acknowledgment of unnecessary technocratic interventions as forms of violence as well as engagement with structural violence/s (Sadler et al., 2016). As a result, birth violence is now defined as including a wider range of 'categories,' including: physical violence, verbal and emotional violence, unnecessary medical technologies, and structural violence embedded in system inadequacies (see Freedman et al., 2014; Bohren et al., 2015; Khosla et al., 2016; Sadler et al., 2016). However, it is still unclear how these multiple aspects or 'categories' of violence are related and how to develop research, advocacy, intervention and implementation strategies to address them (Freedman & Kruk, 2014; Freedman et al., 2014; Jewkes & Penn-Kekana, 2015; Khosla et al., 2016; Sadler et al., 2016). At the moment, birth violence or 'obstetric violence' is ill-defined (Jewkes & Penn-Kekana, 2015) and under-theorized. We thus lack understandings of how different materializations of violence are connected and how they relate to biomedicine, racialized patriarchy, geopolitics and intersectional power relations.

In order to further thinking and action, I argue that we need to move away from individualized readings of birth violence, which are in danger of producing static perpetrator and victim positions (Chadwick, 2017b). We also need to prioritize not only direct and overt forms of physical violence but also explore hidden, normalized and invisible forms of violence. This chapter thus conceptualizes birth violence, not as a narrow interpersonal encounter, but as multiple, shifting, relational, emergent and entangled with a range of sociomaterial forces, discourses, objects, norms and structures. I explore the violations produced and enacted in birth narratives and the ways in which 'gentle' relations of domination targeted, constrained and *generated* laboring/bodies as passive, constricted and diminished. I argue that multiple forms of power intra-act (i.e. biomedical, racialized patriarchy, class) to enact modes of embodied oppression during labor/birth as everyday and 'normal' within particular birth assemblages. I am thus predominantly interested in the normalized and often hidden forms of violence enacted during labor/birth. This chapter thus does not focus on direct or 'hard' physical violence, but tries to 'look sideways' (Žižek, 2008) at the violence that materializes as hidden, normalized and often invisible relations of domination. According to Žižek (2008), it is these invisible forms of violence that create the conditions of possibility for outbreaks of overt physical abuse. A range of terms have been used to refer to these subtle, often imperceptible forms of violence, including: structural (Galtung, 1969), symbolic (Bourdieu, 2001), objective (Žižek, 2008) or 'soft' violence (Colaguori, 2010). Key to all of these conceptualizations is the notion that hidden violences operate beyond individual intentions, choices and pathologies and are embedded in social norms and material relations of domination and power.

Gentle violence

> Actions that compel people to conform to social structures through symbolic power are not neutral exchanges but exchanges that maintain relations of domination.
>
> *(Colaguori, 2010, p. 395)*

Symbolic violence is defined as, "relations and mechanisms of domination and power which do not arise from overt physical force or violence on the body" (Morgan & Thapar-Björkert, 2006, p. 443). These are *hidden* or *invisible* forms of violence that operate via the naturalization and normalization of injustice, powerlessness and violation (Colaguori, 2010). Symbolic violence is thus not necessarily harsh or forceful; rather it, "is a type of submission . . . a gentle violence, imperceptible and invisible even to its victims" (Bourdieu cited in Colaguori, 2010, p. 395). Such invisible forms of 'gentle violence' exert domination via submission, compliance, obedience and acceptance rather than direct coercion or physical force and function as generative sociomaterial forces that intra-actively shape bodies and actions in particular directions (Colaguori, 2010). Normalized violence is also generative in that it contributes to the maintenance and reiteration of hegemonic social relations of power, status, hierarchy and control. It is made up of a constellation of rational and orderly practices, norms and sociomaterial relations that normalize, stabilize and naturalize domination and injustice and enact embodied oppression/s. The following section explores women's birth narratives in/through the concept of 'gentle violence,' exploring how women *became* submissive, passive, docile and compliant body-subjects in the contextual logics of disempowering birth assemblages.

Normalizing powerlessness

Some low-income women enacted positions of passivity without question or complaint. For these women, passivity and powerlessness were 'normal' during labor/birth in MOU settings. They accepted that they were patients, object-bodies and subject to 'orders' and that nurses were experts that dictated the process of labor/birth. Passivity was thus a core subject position or 'way of being' for some low-income women (see Zadoroznyj, 1999). In 'passive' birth stories, there was thus little evidence of self-determination, agency or fleshy embodiment. According to Lyerly (2006, p. 103) agency is "the power and the presence to preside over one's own experience of giving birth." While this is in part a problematic definition rooted in a middle-class ideal of birth in which control over the body is valorized, the idea of presence is useful as a means of thinking about agency as embodied capacity. In stories that enacted passive and muted subjectivities during labor/birth, there was little sense of body or presence. Instead, in these tellings, a sense of absence and powerlessness was pervasive. However, rather than being distressed or dissatisfied about their lack of active agency, some women constructed their powerlessness and passivity as 'normal,' expected, acceptable and unremarkable. Passivity was thus told via a matter-of-fact mode of storytelling. Being dominated by nurses was construed as banal and everyday, with birth enacted as an event in which things were done to them, they were told what to do and where to do it, with little space for agency or iterations of selfhood.

Rachelle: And the nurses? Did you have to call them when you felt the baby was coming?

Waheeda: No, they came to call you.

Rachelle: They were already with you?

Waheeda: No, they came to call me in the labor ward and they um, took me where the, where they give birth, where the ladies give birth—in another room.

Rachelle: Okay, so why did they call you? I'm not following—why did they call you?

Waheeda: Because they told me to put on the gown (R: yes).

Rachelle: Is this after they gave you the injection and the pain got worse?

Waheeda: Yes (laughs)

Rachelle: So then they knew you were ready?

Waheeda: Yes (R: okay, okay) And then they told me just to lay there, just checked the sound, to see if the baby's heart was beating and everything and I was laying there for about half an hour, they told me, "Now come" and they prepared everything for me now to give birth.

(Black, low-income, MOU birth)

In this account, there is little sense of active agency or embodied presence. 'They' (nurses) are the dominant actors: "they came to call you," "they came to call me," "they took me," "they prepared everything for me now to give birth."

Significantly, Waheeda only uses the word "I" once in this exchange and even then it is only to indicate passivity: "I was laying there." Her fleshy laboring/birthing body is absent and there is no reference to her embodied labor sensations, feelings, movements, pains or needs. Waheeda's body is enacted as the passive object of biomedical instructions and its fleshy vitality erased. She never refers to an urge to push or any feeling that delivery was imminent. Instead, 'putting on the gown' and being moved to another room mark the progression of labor instead of her own bodily sensations. Her experience is so dominated by medical others that she is left with little story to tell and is not recognizable as a visible protagonist in her own birth narrative.

As a middle-class interviewer, I found it difficult to 'follow' or understand Waheeda, largely because of her persistent privileging of the nurses' point of view and the absence of the laboring/birthing body in her story. This made no sense to me in the context of narrating a birth experience. In my initial question, I assume Waheeda's positionality as agentic and the laboring body as an active force—i.e. "Did you have to call them when you felt the baby was coming?" Throughout her responses she repeatedly reproduced herself as passive rather than agentic. In the research assemblage, this encounter between me (a white, privileged, middle-class woman) and Waheeda (poor, young, pregnant, black, unemployed and lacking social capital) was full of disconnects and misunderstandings. Given her sociomaterial location, Waheeda was likely familiar with positions of marginality and limited decision-making. As a result, *from her perspective*, passivity was regarded as a normalized and acceptable subject position. According to Young (1990b), powerlessness is a materialization of oppression whereby the socially powerless come to expect to take orders from powerful others and assume positions of subservience. Obedience and passivity thus become normalized in everyday enactments of oppression. There is no need for direct or 'hard' violence to enforce passivity or obedience when relations of domination and oppression are naturalized as 'normal.'

Along with assuming positions of passivity in their birth stories, low-income women utilizing public sector services often did not expect to make choices during labor. For example, many women spoke about being injected with substances and having no idea about what was being put into their bodies. This was, however, accepted as normal and not seen as problematic.

Rachelle:	Did you have any injections?
Bonita:	They, they, it's a new injection (. . .) they gave me two injections, the birth control—the three months—and then they gave another injection, it's a new injection.
Rachelle:	Do they explain what it is?
Bonita:	Uhuuh.
Rachelle:	So you don't know what it was?
Bonita:	That one goes in our backside.
Rachelle:	Okay, did you want the injection?
Bonita:	(★★) They give the injection (R: yes), they give it just like that.

(Black, low-income, MOU birth)

Rachelle: Did they give you any pain relief?

Wendy: The one nurse **did** give me *uuh* (*) *injection*, don't know what kind of injection was in there.

(Black, low-income, MOU transferred to public hospital)

Low-income women often did not know what drugs or injections were being administered to them. Rather than being problematized or regarded as unacceptable, women operated within an understanding that in public sector settings, interventions were not negotiable and there was no space to question or refuse treatments. Passivity and powerlessness thus emerged as product/s of particular birth assemblages in which capacities for agency were disallowed or constrained. Within public sector birth assemblages, individual 'choices' and 'desires' are not enabled or expected. For example, Bonita was clearly nonplussed when she was asked in the interview (see page 106) if she *wanted* the injection and responded, "they give the injection, they give it just like that," indicating that no choice, desire or negotiation was involved. Most low-income women accepted the absence of choice as normal and made no complaints about it. A lack of choice regarding pain relief during labor was also accepted as normative and 'the way things are done' in the public sector. Thus, according to Abigail, "They give nothing for pain" and Bonita, "They give us no pain relief, only when we are <u>finished</u>." Low-income women did not expect to make 'choices' about pain relief or mode of delivery or have their 'desires' recognized or fulfilled. They were also not necessarily upset by the lack of choices available to them but accepted this as the normal order of things.

Performing docility

While some women accepted positions of powerlessness, others were more active and reflexive in their enactments of passivity. Interestingly, several women thus spoke about *actively performing passivity* as a way of negotiating adequate care in local health care settings. Paradoxically, the performance of docility was thus described as a strategy. In the South African context, the notion of the 'good patient' has been identified as a key theme in public sector health services (Khalil, 2009; Schneider et al., 2010) and maternity settings (Jewkes, Abrahams & Mvo, 1998). Nurses have been found to define 'good patients' as obedient, polite, clean and undemanding while 'difficult patients' are seen as rude, aggressive, uncooperative and demanding (Khalil, 2009). In public health care settings, 'good patients' are often rewarded with care, while 'bad' or difficult patients are ignored and do not always get needed medical care. There are therefore potentially serious costs for those that are deemed to be 'difficult.' Public sector patients often make considerable efforts to exert the "expert patient strategy" (Schneider et al., 2010, p. 141) and present themselves as obedient, docile and knowledgeable. In under-resourced Southern contexts more broadly, medical professionals have been found to, "set priorities for who gets available services" (Spangler, 2011, p. 492). Patients who can present themselves as ideal 'good patients' are more likely to receive these services. Given that social inequalities materialize as 'embodied inequalities' (Spangler, 2011), marginalized women are often compromised in health care settings. They struggle to present themselves as 'good patients' given that race, ethnicity, poverty, age, HIV and marital status often mark them as automatically 'bad patients.'

Low-income women were often aware of the importance of presenting themselves as compliant during labor in order to secure adequate treatment from nurses. For example:

Asanda: The treatment was much better in [public hospital] than in [MOU].

Rachelle: How? How was it better?

Asanda: Cause the people are more supporting in [public hospital], more than [MOU], yes.

Rachelle: In what sort of way were they supportive compared to the other?

Asanda: The problem is at [MOU] um (*) the nurses get (**) I dunno how to say it—pissed off very easily and the(y), they get like annoyed, that's the problem there, if you are nagging too much or asking too much then they get like pissed off—I dunno why.

Rachelle: And did that happen to you?

Asanda: This time yes but I was trying to avoid that cause I was also in pain

Rachelle: Okay, so how do you try and avoid them getting angry?

Asanda: Byyyy doing what they say I must do, yes

Rachelle: So being, just kind of listening and being a kind of good #

Asanda: Patient, yes.

(Black, low-income, MOU birth)

Being obedient and performing the role of the docile, 'good patient' emerged as a reflexive strategy some women took up in order to receive care and avoid angry nurses and potential mistreatment. Even while in the midst of a painful labor, Asanda describes self-regulating her behavior to make sure she presented as undemanding and passive. In this way, the 'good patient' ideal functions as a mode of regulation and self-discipline that constructs docile laboring bodies. There is no thus no need for overt physical violence here. Threats of violence and mistreatment circulate as affective currents within MOU settings and are often enough to constrain, control and regulate women's behaviors.

This is symbolic violence, that 'gentle' and non-forceful violence that produces submission and compliance (Colaguori, 2010) or what Foucault would refer to as normalizing or disciplinary power that works to produce docile, self-disciplining subjects. Birth assemblages in public sector MOUs are organized according to the logic of hierarchy, control, normalized expectations of patient passivity and the possibility of punishment (via violence/mistreatment or neglect) for those that do not conform to norms and requirements (see Jewkes, Abrahams & Mvo, 1998). Hierarchical power relations require the enactment of prescribed roles of expert/patient in which the patient willingly becomes a passive and obedient patient-body.

Abigail:	If you just listen to them, they [nurses] are quite fine.
Rachelle:	If you listen?
Abigail:	**Listen** yes, but if you go and do your **own** thing then they will also not stand by you.
Rachelle:	Can you give me an example of what you mean by listen?
Abigail:	Maybe they told you, "Go pee quickly *in that thing*" and then (★) they test now—with a straw and then they say "Go and throw that quickly away for us," "Sit quickly on the bed," "Lie quickly that way," "Lie this way," *soooo . . .*

As Abigail describes, as long as laboring women obeyed orders and did not 'speak back,' the nurses were "fine" and there was no mistreatment, abuse or neglect. As Abigail says, the price of not being obedient is the possible loss of medical care ("they will also not stand by you"). A birth assemblage arranged according to normalized expectations of docility and prescriptive requirements for attaining 'good patient' status, engenders a situation in public sector clinics where some women adopt a "hesitant, docile, silent body" (Shabot, 2016, p. 246) as a way of avoiding mistreatment. Operating according to a logic of hierarchical relations, normalization of mistreatment and abuse (see Jewkes, Abrahams & Mvo, 1998) and the possibility of punitive treatment for failing to enact the 'good patient' script, MOU birth assemblages *produce* docile bodies, passivity and compressed selves. There is limited room for the construction of forms of active agency during birth—or at least forms of agency recognizable within middle-class frameworks. The forms of constricted agency described above constitute modes of 'ambiguous agency' (Geerts & van der Tuin, 2013) in which enactments of passivity and docility can become (constrained) forms of agency. Reflexive enactments of compliance and obedience become paradoxically both active enactments or as argued by Tanassi (2004), a "material strategy" that women perform *and* modes of control, domination and regulation that limit agency and oppress embodied selves. Any agency produced in such assemblages is thus at best 'ambiguous.'

Illusions of 'choice'

Low-income women utilizing public sector services did not expect to be able to exercise choices in relation to mode of birth, pain relief and interventions. Framed by discourses of pregnancy/birth as modes of neoliberal consumption and identity-making and given their access to privatized health care, middle-class women did expect to make choices during labor/birth. For many privileged women that I spoke to, 'choice' was a core ideal in relation to birth. It was seen as imperative that a woman exercises choice in relation to mode of birth, place of birth, type of pain relief (epidural, nitrous gas, pethidine, water birth), the use of birthing accessories (birthing balls, pools, doulas, music) and chosen caregivers and birth companions (partners, relatives, friends, children).

Erin: I mean for me if, if somebody makes an informed choice, that's fine.

(White, homebirth)

Lola: I think it should be your choice, it's your body (*) it's your baby.

(White, elective caesarean)

The perspectives of the privileged women in this study mirror approaches to birth in neoliberal Northern contexts, where birth is increasingly seen as part of a broader 'consumer culture' in which the "choosing self" (Slater cited in Zukin & Maguire, 2004, p. 180) and active consumer (Fannin, 2003) are ideal models of birthing agency (see Chapter 2). While privileged women in South Africa ostensibly have access to an array of choices during pregnancy concerning mode/place of birth and chosen caregivers, the birth experience sometimes proves to be an event in which the promise of choice and agency evaporates. To illustrate, I will use Alison's birth story as a case example.

When I met Alison, a young, white, newly married middle-class woman, she was six months pregnant and in cheerful and excited spirits about having a 'natural' birth at the local private hospital. According to her, the gynaecologist encouraged 'active birth' but advised her to wait until labor and "decide *then*" what kind of pain relief she wanted. Some months later, we met again and spoke about her birth experience. It was a different Alison that I spoke to this time. Distress was etched on/through her body as she talked. She churned with visible tension and agitation as she told me about her 'nightmare birth' in which she ended up having a raft of interventions, including two epidurals, a range of other pharmacological drugs and an emergency caesarean section. While assured of an array of pain relief options by her gynaecologist before the birth, including pethidine, nitrous gas and water birth, during the actual labor all these 'choices' disappeared. When she asked for an epidural after seven hours of labor, it was not forthcoming and no explanation was offered. Instead, all that seemed available was pethidine, which she took as "nothing else seemed available." After nine hours of labor she received an epidural. Labor complications spiralled and things become increasingly chaotic and distressing.

Alison: The gynae kept saying I'm five centimeters and the midwife would check me and say "No, no, no, you're seven, eight centimeters" so I was a bit, in limbo there as well, um, and then (*) my contractions *slowed* (*) and they, they weren't as strong and then they started worrying about that, um, and he, he put something in this drip that (**) (sighs) that makes the contractions stronger, so, and then, her heart rate kept dropping with each contraction (. . .) and it was, it was horrible and then they said, he [gynaecologist] said, maybe, *maybe* I should go for a caesar, you know, it was never "You must go for a caesar" and I said to him, "No," I, I couldn't understand *why*, everything was, I was nine and a half centimeters by this stage and everything was all go, they could feel her head, there was a bit of pressure on her head but that, I mean there will be, um (★) and I couldn't understand why I, they just wouldn't let my body do the rest, why I had to have this extra stuff and (★) and um (★) then her, it happened four times that her heart rate went down like that and then, the midwife who'd been with me the entire time and another one came in (★) um, cause I was struggling and she just looked at me and she said, "I think your baby's worked hard enough now, you need to go (★) for a caesar," <u>I was crying</u>, I just, all I did, I played for about two hours, you know played them for time, to try and not have a caesar and I was in tears and I didn't wanna go through (. . .) because everything was happening and I felt like my body was working and it knew what *to do*, it was, it's *really* disappointing . . .

The birth left Alison deeply distressed. At the time of our second interview, she was on medication for postnatal depression and still suffered nightmares about the birth. Her marriage had suffered and she had not bonded well with her baby. While she was ostensibly given 'choices' during labor and the gynaecologist never directly ordered or 'forced' her to have a caesarean, in this high-tech birth assemblage, biomedical power relations worked via an entanglement of affective flows, machinery, drugs, measurements, risk discourses and authoritative, expert pressure to shape and compel 'choices' in particular directions. Drug interventions, the foetal monitor and a host of medical professionals worked against Alison's desire to let her body do the work of giving birth. In the end, she was emotionally bullied into having a caesarean section, not by an individual, but by an entanglement of sociomaterial and affective forces. Importantly, this biomedical birth assemblage was not just comprised of a static collection of machines, experts and discourses but was vitalized, materialized and energized by affective flows and intensities. The affective currents vitalizing this biomedical birth assemblage materialized intra-actively in the moment that the midwife says, "your baby's worked hard enough now." This comment sparks an array of diffractive and affective consequences. It inaugurates a sharp split between the needs/desires of the mother and the baby and vitalizes a broader interpretive repertoire in which the pregnant woman/body is constructed as antagonistic to the foetus/baby (Fannin, 2003). The comment also enacts Alison as marginal to her own birth experience and erases her pain, struggle and hard work during labor (i.e. it is not her work, it belongs to the baby). It also mobilizes a discourse of maternal selfishness and 'bad mothering' and suggests that Alison is being selfish and needs to put her baby (and its safety) first. Discourses and affects invoking biomedical risk/safety, selfless/selfish mothering and separation between mother/baby flash and fizz in this encounter, working to intra-actively disable agency and 'choice.' Alison is left in distress with tears streaming down her face and kept repeating in the interview that she still has no idea why, "they wouldn't let my body do the rest." In the end, she 'decides' to have the caesarean.

According to Crossley (2007), Alison's birth story is typical of many middle-class women's experiences of medicalized birth in the Global North. Many privileged women expect to be able to exert agency and choices during labor and have a 'natural' drug-free birth if they so desire. The reality of what happens during birth, when medical professionals hold authoritative knowledge and operate in assemblages dominated by biomedical risk discourses, technoscience and expertise that is vitalized and charged with affective power, is often very different. As Crossley notes (2007, p. 558), "Faced with these 'options'—safe birth/ potential death—how can we be said to be making a choice?" While the 'choices' women and their partners face during labor often become impossibly constrained, neoliberal, consumer discourses continue to construct them (particularly mothers) as ultimately responsible for what kind of birth they experience. Thus, if women do not 'succeed' at having a natural birth or at breastfeeding, they have 'failed' at mothering (see Crossley, 2007) due to some defect, weakness, lack of preparation or questionable determination (Mardorossian, 2003). At the same time as material, technocratic, 'real-life' events in medicalized encounters unfold according to the vocabularies and affective currents of risk, safety, authoritative expertise, selfless mothering and parental responsibility, middle-class women are also prepped to believe that they can exercise choices and be active agents during labor. Is it therefore surprising that many women are left torn between a range of conflicting and irreconcilable emotions during and after medicalized birth? According to Alison, her birth contravened all her expectations and was experienced as 'traumatic.'

Alison: I didn't feel like it was, it was *me*, it kind of went against my (*) my *ideal* and the person I thought I was, do you know what I, like (R: ja) like your mom did it like this and there's like no reason why you *can't* (R: hmm, hmm) and (*) and my body was doing all the right things, but it, it just wasn't allowed to (*) finish the, the job . . .

Alison assumed that birth would reflect or confirm her identity or 'ideal self.' As she mentioned in the pre-birth interview, she felt that giving birth would make her, "feel bigger afterwards," proud, enlarged and confident. Instead she was left feeling depressed, distressed and diminished. A key aspect of this diminishment was that her body was not 'allowed' to fulfil its own capacities or do the work of giving birth. While there was no direct violence, coercion or domination here, the affective and relational landscape of the birth assemblage evoked a sense of diminishment and powerlessness. Instead of working to enhance Alison's sense of bodily capacity and involvement in the process of giving birth, health care providers worked against her laboring body. Nearly fully dilated and feeling as if her body "was working and it knew what *to do*," she was 'gently coerced' into having a caesarean section without an adequate explanation or justification why it was necessary. She was left feeling that her birth experience contravened her sense of self and bodily agency and "the person I thought I was."

'Gentle violence' thus produced passive, mute/d and constrained laboring/ birthing bodies without the need for overt violence or force. For several low-income women, passivity was a 'normal' subject position. For other women, the threat of violence, neglect and mistreatment was enough to ensure *enactments* of obedience and docility. In privatized, private sector birth assemblages, women's choices and agency were at times erased by an intra-active entanglement of experts, machines and circuits of affective and relational intensities vitalized by discourses of risk and 'good' mothering. Compliance and submission were thus produced, not by direct or overt violence, but within/through the structuring logics of birth assemblages and affective circuits of biomedical and gendered power relations.

Embodied oppression/s

In addition to 'gentle' modes of violence, women who did not conform to 'good patient' ideals, either because of their 'unruly' behavior or because they were 'marked' as problematic by their sociomaterial locations (i.e. poor, young, unmarried, multiparous, HIV+) became the direct targets of bodily disciplining and punishment, particularly in MOU settings. Women's laboring/birthing bodies, as (potentially threatening) fleshy enactments of agency, power and difference, became the sites of normalized relational violence, which worked to constrain and punish. As I explore below, many women were subjected to modes of 'embodied oppression' (Shabot, 2016) during labor/birth that worked to suppress, discipline and reduce their bodily selves, fleshy corporeality and 'embodied agency.'

Constraining embodied agency

'Agency' should not be thought of in a disembodied manner as the freedom to make choices and decisions. Particularly in relation to birth, agency is deeply embodied and involves the freedom to follow, engage with and negotiate the psychofleshy challenges of labor. As I have argued previously (see Chapter 2), biomedicine frames birthing bodies as pure physiology split off from the emotional and subjective complexity of embodied personhood (Sbisà, 1996; Goldberg, 2002). The ideal medical body is an inanimate, object body and not the lived, embodied self. According to Leder (1992, p. 117), modern medicine is founded upon a metaphysics based on "the dead, inanimate body" and seeks to transform the energetic force of the embodied self into "corpse-like passivity" (p. 121). The distinction made by Merleau-Ponty between the lived body (*Leib*) and physical body (*Körper*) is pertinent here (see Shabot, 2016). In obstetrics, there is often a tension between the ideal, passive biomedical body (*Körper*) and the body-in-labor (*Leib*), which is an active, powerful and forceful corporeality.

Shabot (2016) argues that violence in the birthing room is fundamentally different from other forms of medical violence because the laboring body is usually "a healthy and powerful body" (p. 2) that is also deeply sexual. This exuberant body threatens both the ideal of the passive, biomedical object-body and normative modes of feminine embodiment. Mistreatment during birth can thus function as modes of gender and medical discipline that constrain and punish the 'loud,' powerful force of the laboring and birthing body (see Shabot, 2016). When applied to the lively, pulsating, generative and fleshy body that births, the routine practices of medicine (objectification, treating the body as passive *Körper*) become particularly problematic and potentially harmful. As a result, being treated as a passive, depersonalized body that is only there to be manipulated, monitored and practiced upon, has been linked to distressing experiences of birth and the development of birth trauma (Beck, 2004, 2009). Importantly, being able to enact forms of embodied agency, in which self/body are enmeshed in meaningful modes of connection during labor, has been found to be a critical component of positive birth experiences (Akrich & Pasveer, 2004).

While some poor women managed to find ways of constructing forms of embodied agency during labor, others had their efforts to enact forms of bodily agency constantly interrupted. The affective matrix in which birth unfolded was a key force shaping women's bodily capacities and their ability to enact forms of embodied agency during labor. For example:

Kuhle: So around past two I feel like (★) if I push there's {something coming} so **I was**, there in my bed there's a, a chart, there's two charts, so I was sitting there, and when I'm sitting there I feel like, if I open my, my legs (R: hmm) I feel comfortable, so I open my legs (★) so then the sister came and check and she said, "Why are you doing this?" I said, "I feel like to do this thing" she said, "No, it's not a good thing" I said "Okay," I stand up and then I go to the bed and I take the other cushions and put them on top and then I just feel like this.

Rachelle: What did they want you to do?

Kuhle: They say, they said I must sleep, I must sleep.

Rachelle: You must sleep? Flat on back?

Kuhle: Ja [yes], back flat ja, so I don't feel like it (R: hmm) I just feel like to do that thing I want to do (R: hmm) ok then, after that I said "I want to push" they said "No, don't push, you are not allowed to push—you must go to that side," I said, "Okay," I go to that side and then, so when I go to the other side, they check me there, blood and then they checked the heartbeat of the baby and they said "It's fine" so I asked, "Can I push now?" they said, "<u>No</u>, wait," I push myself because they said, "<u>No</u>, don't push" but *I feel like* (R: you want to?) yes, so I push and then they are shouting, "Sissie [sister], why are you pushing? I said don't push!" I said, "I feel like I want to push," they said, "<u>**No**</u>! I didn't say *push*!" (inaudible) so I rather keep quiet . . .

(Black, low-income, MOU birth)

Kuhle tries to follow her embodied sensations and do what feels comfortable in the midst of the painful, fleshy labor experience. Instead of enabling and supporting her bodily urges, health care providers constantly interrupt her efforts to enact embodied agency. Birth evokes powerful forms of embodiment in which women are confronted by the force/pain of contractions and the manifestation of a new mode of corporeality that cannot easily be denied. This is the 'body-in-labor' described as a "pendulum movement" in which the body swings between the presence and absence of overwhelming and violent pain during contractions (Akrich & Pasveer, 2004, p. 68).

Akrich and Pasveer (2004) argue that the experience of labor is one of fundamental duality involving two central bodily actors, namely: the body-in-labor and the embodied self. The forms of (dis)connection and (dis)association that women negotiate between these two forms of embodiment is key to determining whether birth is experienced as empowering or disempowering. When raw, bodily sensations and external factors (measurements, expectations, assessments of health care providers) match, women are able to construct forms of body–self connection and association. When these do not match, there is possible disconnection, loss of meaning and the objectification of the body-in-labor (Akrich & Pasveer, 2004). An alienated experience of birth is described as one in which the duality between the two forms of embodiment (body-in-labor and embodied self) are obliterated, "either because the body-in-labor is too present and takes over, or because it is absent" (p. 80). In Kuhle's case, she is caught between efforts to construct embodied agency by following raw bodily sensations (taking up bodily positions that feel viscerally comfortable; feeling the urge to push) and listening to nurses who constantly invalidate her bodily sensations. Repeatedly told that she cannot trust or follow the urges of the body-in-labor, she is left split *between* external medical orders, instructions and requirements and her own powerful bodily feelings. She is shouted at and scolded for trying to enact forms of embodied agency and has to get 'permission' from nurses before she is 'allowed' to push. Nurses deny and invalidate the powerful psychofleshy experience of labor/birth and Kuhle's privileged access to bodily feelings, knowledge and sensations. Ironically, at the same time, medical posters in this birth assemblage encourage women to adopt active birthing positions. Kuhle is, however, punished when she tries to follow their suggestions.

Kuhle: They, they put the pictures there, if you are in labor you are supposed to do this and that but when I am doing this, they say, "No, it's not allowed."

Contradictory messages about laboring bodies thus abound in this birth assemblage. While medical posters advocate evidence-based practices such as encouraging women to adopt active birth/labor positions (i.e. squatting), this is disallowed by health care providers who insist that Kuhle adopt an outdated and harmful method of delivery (i.e. the supine position). Rather than supporting or facilitating women's 'loud bodies' (Shabot, 2016) and psychofleshy experience during labor/birth, low-income women repeatedly told stories in which health care professionals tried to control, punish and 'mute' exuberant and assertive displays of embodied agency and laboring corporeality. The ontological assumptions of obstetric knowledge/practice that birth is a medical event and that the laboring body is *Körper*, a depersonalized, passive, purely physiological object of medical knowledge and treatment, were thus vitalized and enacted in this everyday MOU encounter. While objects countering normative assumptions (i.e. posters) circulated as part of this assemblage, disempowering ontological frames continued to dominate, shaping the ways in which nurses treated and interacted with women during labor/birth.

In women's stories, the bodily process of birth was enacted as a source of frustration for nurses as they struggled to maintain control in the delivery room. Fadwah, for example, was reprimanded and punished simply for involuntary bodily movements during delivery.

Fadwah: And um like I was pushing, I was moving on the bed because of the plastic that was on the bed and **I didn't notic**e I was moving, like she told me I must lay straight (*) and I didn't know that I was like moving (*) and then **she shouts** and then she say, "Lay straight, why are you laying that way?" (cross voice).

(Black, low-income, MOU birth)

This nurse felt compelled to punish Fadwah for being an 'unruly' body that refused to 'lay straight.' Her birthing body, active and exuberant, had to be disciplined and regulated to conform to normative and hierarchical relations of medical and class power, where the nurse is supposed to be the expert with status and the (black and poor) birthing woman is supposed to be the passive, stigmatized and obedient body-object. At the same time, because power relations in birth assemblages are never fixed and are continually emergent processes, nurses can feel compelled to continually reassert control over the birth process and discipline 'unruly' and 'loud' birthing bodies. In obstetric assemblages structured by a logic of hierarchical punishment and control, the volatility and unpredictability of the laboring body can become a problem or threat that needs to be contained. For Shabot (2016), the noisy birthing body is a threat to norms of feminine passivity and docility. The stories of low-income black women show that norms pertaining to 'good femininity' are embedded in racialized power relations. As a result, poor black women were often punished for being 'loud' and screaming during birth via accusations of sexual promiscuity or lasciviousness (see extracts on page 122). Women's loud and unruly birthing bodies also potentially disrupt medical norms and ideals of the 'good patient' body. As a result of the disruptive potential of the fleshy birthing body to challenge multiple sociomaterial and medicalized norms pertaining to 'good bodies,' punishing women via verbal abuse, rough treatment and forms of relational violence is sometimes sanctioned and normalized by medical staff and authorities (see Bohren et al., 2016).

While some women had their efforts to construct forms of embodied agency disallowed in/through relational exchanges with nurses, other women in the public sector spoke about technology and machines as objects of frustration that constrained their embodied agency during labor. For example:

Madiha:	**I ask, I ask**, I ask them—can't they just make this thing *looser* because the pain comes at the back and <u>that thing</u> is ↑*tight, tight, tight*↑ and then they said "<u>No</u>, that thing is because the baby's heart, to monitor the baby's heart and that."
Rachelle:	So it was very uncomfortable for you?
Madiha:	{*Very*, very uncomfortable}
Rachelle:	And did you lie on the bed—you didn't walk up and down?
Madiha:	**There was**, I couldn't even walk <u>because</u> {*the drips are all here in my hands*}
Rachelle:	Oh you couldn't walk—would you have preferred to #
Madiha:	I would have liked to have walked because when you get pains you couldn't sit up ↑you couldn't lie on your back↑ because that thing then *makes* another, then he **scratches** so and stuff (R laughs) *that thing* that does that man, he <u>scratches</u> the whole time on the page, now you can't lie on your back, you have to lie on your side the whole time so that, <u>that thing</u> can (★) monitor (★) the baby (R: okay, okay)
Rachelle:	So the machines weren't very nice?
Madiha:	*You couldn't move*, you had to just lie *the whole time* on your side, <u>this side</u> already went lame.

(Black, low-income, public hospital birth)

Madiha is frustrated because she is constrained by an electronic foetal monitor (EFM), animated in her story as "that thing" and an intravenous drip. She is unable to walk, sit up or move during labor because of "that thing," which adds considerably to her discomfort and pain. Obstetric technology in this scenario is vitalized as an agentic force that adds to suffering and disallows embodied agency. Her request to have the EFM loosened is refused, communicating that the machine is more important than her feelings of comfort. This is a disempowering materialization of obstetric technology in which the machine is valorized over the laboring woman and used to constrain and objectify rather than as a means of establishing possible body–self connectivity. According to Lyerly (2006), obstetric technology is not inherently disempowering; instead, it intra-acts with other forces in the assemblage to affect women in different ways. Sensitively applied with/in an affirming relational matrix, obstetric interventions, "can actually enhance a woman's ability to engage more fully in her birthing experience" (p. 112). In Madiha's case, the machine is entangled with/in wider relational, discursive and affective currents of biomedical objectification and the valorization of technology, resulting in the diminishment of agency and lack of body–self connectivity.

Exposure and loss of dignity

'Dignity' has been identified by patients as the second most important aspect of health care, following access to services (Jacobson, 2007). It has been defined as a principle asserting the inherent value that belongs to each person on the basis of their basic humanity (Jacobson, 2007). However, dignity is not just an abstract principle but is thoroughly relational, embodied and gendered. It is affirmed or violated in the everyday social relations between persons, institutions, technologies and sociosymbolic structures. In relation to birth, maintaining dignity is intertwined with the respectful treatment of the laboring/birthing body and the maintenance of privacy. As discussed in Chapter 4, fear of loss of dignity during birth often involves concerns about having the deeply private and eroticized genital zone open for viewing, objectification and interference during labor/birth. Privileged women thus worried about the loss of dignity and control that would come from the exposure of their most private and intimate body parts during birth (see Chapter 4). These narratives suggested that the maintenance of bodily privacy is of key importance to many women during birth. While privacy has been recognized as a difficult concept to define, essentially it involves our rights as persons to be free from unwanted intrusions and to maintain control over our personal physical space and bodily integrity. Birth is a time of vulnerable corporeality in which bodily boundaries are destabilized and fluid, and 'private' zones become potentially exposed, without consent or control, to outside others. While privileged women were scared of the risks of being exposed and losing bodily dignity during birth, dignity and privacy violations materialized as realities in the birth stories of low-income, black women. In these stories, dignity violations were narrated as unwanted *exposures* of both self and body in which privacy (i.e. bodily privacy and privacy of personal information) were violated.

Poor women described violations of bodily privacy during labor/birth, in which intimate parts of their bodies were exposed to strangers and they had to endure having their personal bodily zone invaded. For example, Tracy-Lee spoke about the tendency for curtains around labor beds to be left open in MOUs, which resulted in women-in-labor being visually exposed to strangers. As Tracy-Lee said, "it's like <u>no privacy</u>, I can look at the next woman <u>right next to me</u> and I'm here with my partner so there's no privacy, it's really disgusting." For Tracy-Lee, pregnant with her first baby, it was frightening and traumatic to witness how other women were treated during labor and their bodies exposed. For example:

Tracy-Lee:	The way they treat them [laboring women], it's like ↑"Co(me), come, you wanted this, you wanted to have the child—*push, push!* Hold your legs↑" and **forcing** the legs open, like one keep this one and the one keep that way . . .
Rachelle:	So you had to see this?
Tracy-Lee:	I saw this yes, cause I was laying on the bed, sometimes they don't close the curtains and then anybody can come in there, like while the people are giving birth and then I actually had to stand up and while they were writing in my maternity record book and I had to <u>see</u> this happening (**) cause it's like, the beds is all open (R: hmm, hmm)
Rachelle:	I mean that is traumatizing . . .
Tracy-Lee:	**It is**! It's scary!

Rachelle: Especially when it's your first baby . . .

Tracy Lee: Yes, and it was *scary*, I was really, I was really afraid, I thought I'd rather give birth at home than suffer like that (★★) I just wanted to come home, I actually *cried* when my family came to visit and I was like: "Please take me home."

(Black, low-income, MOU labor transferred to public hospital)

Women were thus left unprotected from violations of their bodily privacy and intrusions into their intimate, private zone (i.e. "anybody can come in there"). With curtains left open, laboring and birthing women were subject to the gaze of any random passer-by (medical staff, cleaners, other women in labor and their partners/companions). As Vanessa said, "there is no privacy, I look at you and you look at me." Because she was transferred to a hospital, Tracy-Lee was able to contrast the lack of bodily privacy in the MOU with the respect for privacy that was afforded to women in the public hospital setting.

Rachelle: Did you have someone else in the room with you? [at public hospital]

Tracy-Lee: Yes, there was six of us, it was a very nice experience because everybody was treated, everybody was talking about the nice experience they were having there.

Rachelle: And was there a bit more privacy?

Tracy-Lee: Everything. And every time they check you, even if it's just like to feel your heartbeat, they close the curtains (R: okay, okay) much better, yes.

Low-income women were also faced with violations of privacy in relation to the exposure of private and sensitive information. For example, Jasmine, severely impoverished and pregnant with her third baby, deliberately did not go to the local maternity clinic for antenatal care because she wanted to avoid talk and gossip about her 'situation.' This situation included extreme impoverishment. Jasmine and her three children lived in a dilapidated back room, filled with holes and leaks, which left them exposed to the weather, and with no furniture apart from a bed. Her most recent boyfriend had abandoned her, she was being physically abused by her brothers, was a recovering drug addict, had no income and had recently tried to commit suicide. All of these personal issues, which she referred to as "house problems" were known by local community members. While she managed to avoid the clinic during pregnancy and during birth (she gave birth at home with no birth attendant), Jasmine and her newborn baby did go to the clinic after the birth for a check-up. Nurses then used knowledge of her personal situation to try and coerce her into being sterilized.

Rachelle: So you didn't go to the clinic for health care during your pregnancy?

Jasmine: No, I didn't.

Rachelle: Because they were going to say things about you?

Jasmine:	Yes.
Rachelle:	The nurses or others?
Jasmine:	The nurses also because my [relative] used to work at the MOU and if there's house problems here then they will *talk* together (R: okay) and the night I was supposed to be discharged 11 o' clock, so the nurse told me she knows about the house problems and I was a little bit angry because (inaudible) and they said I must stand by the table, so I thought they're gonna, because supposedly I have to get discharged at 11 o' clock and the one sister said "No, she was supposed to go home at 11 o' clock but her [relative] said she can't go because she's a problem child, she make trouble" and that, and I didn't talk, just my body language wasn't right, that why I didn't say anything and the sterilize story also—they said they're gonna send me to sterilize me, I wouldn't have said anything but there was a lot of sisters and everyone was *staring* at me, so I said, "Sister, I'm not going because sister I didn't say, I didn't sign for it," it's almost like they're wanting to force, force, force.

(Black, low-income, unplanned homebirth)

Jasmine was deeply ashamed of her poverty and did not want it to become further exposed at the health care clinic. As she put it, "what are people gonna say if *I* uh (*) gonna *give birth* like that." It was because of fear of exposure and shaming that she decided to give birth at home with no caregiver and did not attend antenatal care during pregnancy. Poverty is a substantial source of shame for women and is often associated with moral pathology (Adair, 2002) and being a 'bad patient' or 'bad mother.' As a result, the fear of exposure, stigmatization and public shaming can impact on health-seeking behavior and result in some women avoiding health care institutions. Sociomaterial inequalities become 'embodied inequalities' during birth as poverty is inscribed, via social exclusions, onto the bodies of poor women. Women without baby supplies, nappies and clothes bear the very real corpomaterial marks of poverty and are prone to being shamed at health care facilities, labelled as 'bad mothers' and neglected by caregivers (Spangler, 2011). Spangler (2011, p. 491) argues: "Socioeconomic inequalities make their way into women's bodies through multilevel processes of social exclusion that determine the care they can access—their care-seeking behaviour and the treatment they receive."

Women's right to dignifed care, in which they are protected from having the most intimate zones of their bodies and private aspects of their selves exposed, are thus subject to violation in South African public sector services. These violations are not necessarily the result of bad 'intentions' on the part of individual health care providers. Far more ominously, perhaps, they are products of racialized patriarchal and biomedical framings of the body that births, which enact laboring bodies as passive flesh and object-bodies and that deny the embodied subjectivity, personhood and dignity of birthing women. It is only within racialized/patriarchal/

biomedicalized frames that treating women as exposable bodies open to viewing during some of the most intimate and vulnerable moments of their lives could ever be 'normalized.' This is because biomedical and phallocentric ontologies do not recognize the complex intertwining of self, sexuality, flesh, consciousness, power and intimacy that is dispersed in/as the body that births. A drastic shift in the onto-logical conceptualization of birth and birthing bodies is required to address these kinds of everyday and normalized violations. Women should not have to forego their rights to bodily privacy and risk invasion and exposure of their personal zones when giving birth.

Circuits of shame

Public sector birth assemblages were sociomaterial spaces in which bodily shame was often reinforced. Shame is a form of emotional suffering caused by, "the dis-tressed apprehension of the self as inadequate or diminished" (Bartky, 1990, p. 86). According to Sedgwick (1993, p. 12), shame is, "a bad feeling attaching to what one is." In patriarchal cultures, shame is sharply gendered and manifests as a "perva-sive sense of personal inadequacy" (Bartky, 1990, p. 85) and/or via materializations of embodied shame (i.e. unwanted sexual objectification, sexual abuse, cultural dis-gust for women's reproductive bodies). Shame is the affective outcome of finding oneself (or imagining oneself) to be defective and unworthy. Recent studies have argued that many women "organize their personal sense of self around feelings of shame" (Manion, 2003, p. 24). Gendered shame is closely linked to phallocen-tric framings of women's sexual and reproductive bodies as monstrous, repugnant, excessive, contaminating and dirty. Lyerly (2006) argues that the experience of birth, in which women become vulnerable bodies, often exposed and dependent on others for care and support, is a critical locus for understanding gendered shame. Women bring to birth, "a lifetime of experiences relating to the shame of female embodiment" (p. 111). However, gender is, "always over-layered with other cat-egorizations such as class and race" (Skeggs, 1997, p. 115) and gendered modes of bodily shame intersect with class and race to potentially intensify experiences of shame for low-income, black women.

In the public sector, poor and black women were prone to being treated as shameful and 'dirty' in the maternity ward.

Sanele: And then when I get inside [MOU] some of them was not, was not nice with me (★★) they said (★) I must **just go** and (★★) change my, change my, my gowns and that and start to wash **again** because (★★) I have a (★) ↑*stinky*↑(★) <u>smell</u>, so which is, which I don't like because I wake up in the morning <u>here</u> [home] and wash myself because I know alright I am going to the clinic, ↑*so*↑, I was suspicious when I came back, they said I must go and wash because (★) {*I have a smell*}

(Black, low-income, MOU birth)

Roxanne: Then the sisters came who work in the morning but that sister that was with me was **rude** <u>with me</u> (★) because I hadn't brushed my teeth and then she said I mustn't talk in her *face* because my mouth <u>stinks</u> and I must also not throw my clothes on the floor, but I put my clothes <u>neatly</u> on the floor because there wasn't a chair that I could put them on (R: hmm) then she asked me—"Are you so <u>messy</u> at home too?"

(Black, low-income, MOU birth)

Both of these women are confronted with unwelcome images of themselves as 'stinky,' dirty and 'messy.' These kinds of relational exchanges are petty aggressions and humiliations that threaten women's dignity, positive sense of self and generate feelings of being tainted, dirty and inadequate. Women's talk was also saturated with a pervasive sense of being morally judged, blamed and negatively evaluated simply for being a pregnant, black, low-income woman in public health services. The fact that pregnancy was evidence of sexual activity seemed to mark all birthing women in public clinic contexts as potentially 'guilty bodies.' Nurses often shamed women for their sexual activity while they were in crying out in pain or suffering through contractions.

Khule: Then when you're screaming, they say, "No, man, don't make a noise, because the time when you were making a baby you were not screaming, so why are you screaming now?"

(MOU birth)

Sanele: They keep on shouting, the other ones, "You must not assist *her*, is her fault, yo(u), you were not there when she was *having sex* so now <u>she's pregnant</u>, she want your assistance, she must try for herself," they say so.

(MOU birth)

Constance: I screamed because it was <u>burning</u> and she said, the one sister, "No, shut your mouth, why are you screaming? You people keep on screaming because you want to . . ." (★)—wait now—^^"Yes, you people keep on screaming^^ because you want to do such things" and then I said, "But it's sore sister!" then she said, "No, then you mustn't do such things" and then I said, "But I already said sorry to the other sister."

(MOU birth)

In these extracts, low-income and black pregnant women's bodies are enacted as guilty because they have engaged in sexual activity. Bizarrely, one woman (see Constance above) even felt that she needed to 'apologize' to one of the nurses for the fact that she had engaged in sex. The assumption underlying these comments is that poor women should not be having sex or babies and that nurses are responsible for moral policing. Furthermore, the act of giving birth is infused with shaming sexualized innuendos in which women are constructed as deserving of pain and suffering because of suspected lasciviousness, sexual activities and appetites. These kinds of remarks are entangled with longstanding patriarchal/colonial/racist myths and representations that construct black women's sexuality as inherently morally corrupt, and birth pain as women's punishment for wrongdoing. Racialized patriarchal ideas about black women's bodies and sexuality as dangerous, polluting and deserving of punishment are thus reenacted in the birth scene. These 'ideas' materialize vitally as abusive comments that have affective consequences—i.e. they make women feel 'bad' and guilty for being pregnant and reinforce bodily shame linked to women's sexual and reproductive bodies.

Interwoven with comments and actions that reinforced associations between pregnancy and shameful sexual activity was also a devaluation and denigration of birth and women's laboring/birthing bodies as 'dirty' and 'messy.' For example:

Fadwah: I messed on the floor (*) with the blood (R: mhmm) because I was pushing (short laugh), she was there in the office (. . .) now I was messing and she told me um, um, "Go and fetch a mop and clean up your mess" she told me so and I was just looking at her . . .

(Black, low-income, MOU birth)

Asking women to clean up their 'mess' during labor is enabled and entangled with/in sociosymbolic ideas that the laboring body is dirty, polluting and disgusting (Chadwick & Foster, 2013). It also enacts/reflects sociocultural disrespect for birth and triggers a circuit of affective currents that potentially produce visceral feelings of shame in laboring women. Patriarchal frames and languages of birth that reproduce laboring and birthing bodies as monstrous, abject and dirty (see Chapter 4) thus circulate within birth assemblages in unpredictable ways, intra-acting with racialized and classed ideologies, structural conditions and individual persons, to intermittently result in shaming eruptions that frame black women's bodies as guilty, bad, dirty and shameful. Birth assemblages thus potentially become 'circuits of shame' in which (black) women's laboring bodies are read through the languages of racialized patriarchy and class. Given the emergent and heterogeneous nature of assemblages, however, shaming is intermittent and unpredictable. Acts of shaming during labor/birth also need to be understood in the context of wider social configurations of power rather than as the intentional, 'bad' actions of an individual perpetrator. Gendered and racialized body shaming is not just the outcome of an isolated or specific episode but is an integral element of patriarchal ensembles (Bartky, 1990). Birth does not occur outside of gendered, classed and racialized social relations.

Denying embodied personhood

A further aspect of embodied oppression that materialized in women's birth narratives was the denial of embodied personhood. By 'embodied personhood' I mean recognizing the woman-in-labor as a person (with embodied needs and feelings) rather than viewing her simply as a body or passive object. Recognizing women's personhood during labor/birth also means valuing and respecting birth as a significant and personal life event. In low-income women's stories, there were repeated instances in which their status as embodied persons with feelings, needs and rights were denied. Often it was the *structural relations* in clinic/hospital settings that acted to invalidate basic human needs. For example, many women spoke about how they received no food or drink after giving birth to their babies. Some were left hungry after enduring a long and tiring labor and were offered no food at all.

Rachelle: And did you get any food or tea or anything?
Fadwah: No.
Rachelle: Would you have liked something?
Fadwah: <u>Yes</u>! (laughs) after I gave birth (. . .) like as I was, as I was laying there with the baby waiting now for my parents to come (★) I was *hungry* and *thirsty* also (★) and um, that when I asked security if I can't go home because I'm hungry (R: mhmm).

(*Black, low-income, MOU birth*)

According to Vanessa, "a person gets nothing, nothing (. . .) not even a cup of tea or a piece of bread." Given the poverty of many of the women receiving maternity care at public sector institutions, it seems callous that often no effort is made to give women some basic food or offer them tea/coffee to drink, particularly after *giving birth*. Sarayda, talking about the treatment of women during antenatal care visits, criticized the lack of empathy/care shown to pregnant women who were often poor and hungry.

Sarayda: . . . some ladies, you can see they come from a poor background, or you know, things like that, <u>but they're pregnant</u>, and then they even treat that ladies like (★★) like worse, like *look* at you, I mean everybody's situation is different you know, some people come there, women, they're *hungry*, you can see they've got nothing to eat, I used to put in extra food because I know there's always somebody that's hungry and then I share and that.

(*Black, low-income, public hospital*)

The sociomaterial realities of the lives of pregnant women in the public sector are often disregarded by institutional norms, procedures and everyday practices. There seems to be an over-arching lack of recognition (or care) that many pregnant and birthing women are poor and that many cannot afford to bring their own food and supplies. There is thus sometimes no food available, even for women who have been in labor for many hours. As a result, some women are destined to 'suffer' with hunger as Tracy-Lee describes below.

Tracy-Lee: There's a lack of um pillows, there's no pillows at all, you had to sleep on your arm or bring your own pillows, they don't give you food there (★) no food, only in the morning coffee, of which they've got two cups that <u>all the patients</u> must *share* (R: Oh my goodness!) and there's about (★) six beds in the *uuh,* <u>maternity</u> room and then there's eight beds in the postnatal ward and there's only two cups that people must share in the morning and that's only people that's staying there and they give you two <u>dry</u> biscuits with that, the other time you must bring your own food otherwise you're gonna *suffer* (★) and then there's a lack of blankets also, there was only about three of us that had blankets and the girl next to me she was in labor and she had to give me the blanket because I was getting so cold and she closed me with her blanket and she was in labor and looking after me (★) and then next, nobody still came (★) everybody [nurses] was busy skelling [scolding] and things like that.

(MOU transferred to public hospital)

Tracy-Lee paints a dismal picture of public health services during birth in this account. In her version of events, women are left suffering, hungry and without basic items such as pillows and blankets. Women often have to turn to each other for some basic humanity and care. Further disregard for basic human dignity was also evident in the unsatisfactory environment in which many women were expected to labor/birth. Both Vanessa and Tracy-Lee talked about being upset by the dirty and unhygienic conditions women were expected to endure in clinic settings.

Rachelle: And at [MOU]—how was the treatment?
Vanessa: They weren't rude to me, they weren't rude but they just don't care about the people, so (★) and the way the *toilets* look is <u>disgusting</u>, so (★) and when they talk about hygienic, I don't know ***where*** but there's nothing to wash your hands with, nothing, the stuff is *empty* and so . . .

(Black, low-income, MOU birth)

Tracy-Lee: There was one lady [woman-in-labor] who couldn't take the pain, they didn't help her nothing, they just told her to walk if off and her water broke in the toilet and it was laying there till the next morning and that was past 12 at night and it lay there till the next morning and there was a cleaner on duty, but it wasn't cleaned up, it was left there in the toilet and blood stains and things like that, it was really <u>disgusting</u> (R: okay) especially the toilets, it's <u>disgusting</u>, the toilet pots they are cleaned like once a day, the shower—*uurgh!* I don't wanna talk about it, I *uh* didn't wash ***there***, as long as I was laying there I refused to wash there, it was <u>disgusting</u>.

(Black, low-income, MOU transferred to public hospital)

In these birthing scenes women are left hungry, without blankets or pillows and subject to dirty and unhygienic conditions. This is indicative of 'structural disrespect' (Sadler et al., 2016) in which sociomaterial conditions communicate, produce and reflect institutional disregard for pregnant and birthing women. Shaped by sociomaterial and structural forms of disregard and disrespect, such assemblages normalize violating relations and the erasure of women's embodied personhood. Structural disrespect is a sticky logic borne of sociomaterial inequalities that permeates and territorializes (public sector) birth assemblages in South Africa. It is a form of structural violence against women that is normalized and often hidden from view/recognition. However, while these kinds of structural violations often remain invisible as a form of violence, they have powerful visceral and affective consequences. For example, subjected to inhumane conditions during birth (dirty, unhygienic and lacking basic food and blankets) left Tracy-Lee feeling dehumanized and as she put it, "*like an animal.*"

The structuring of sociomaterial space, norms, practices and relations thus often communicated institutional and social disregard, enacting laboring women as unworthy, disposable and without rights to basic dignity (i.e. privacy and embodied personhood). Biomedicalized understandings of laboring bodies as depersonalized objects produced further entanglements in which women were disregarded as embodied persons. For example:

Rachelle: And did you *feel* alone?

Madiha: <u>Very alone</u> because every time one came in [nurse] <u>then they look like that</u> (★★) then **off** they go again, then I said, "<u>Sister</u>, the baby {*is going to come now*}"—"*No*, it's, it's not your first baby man ↑why are you <u>carrying on</u> so?↑"—off they go (..) they were not there in the room where I was alone (R: ok, ok) every time somebody came in {*then they wrote*} then off they go again, *sooo* . . .

(Black, low-income, public hospital birth)

Madiha is muted as an embodied person in this encounter and rendered paradoxically both visible and invisible in the wider swirl of sociomaterial and affective relations. She is treated purely a biomedical body—i.e. as passive flesh to be examined, prodded and assessed. Nurses look and write notes and "then off they go again" without any recognition of her as an embodied person with feelings, anxieties and needs. Thus, while Madiha becomes 'visible' in this encounter as a biomedical body, she is simultaneously rendered invisible as an embodied person. Such muting of patients as embodied selves is not uncommon in biomedical practices more broadly. However, the tendency to see and treat women giving birth as pure object-bodies is particularly disturbing given that they are not 'ordinary' (sick, diseased or injured) patients but vital, psychofleshy embodied selves engaged in a profound and significant life event—i.e. they are giving birth to *new life*.

The tendency to erase women's personhood during medical encounters was not unique to public sector services. Privileged women having elective caesareans also described feeling disregarded and nullified by their experiences in private sector hospitals. For example:

Carrie: So they [husband and baby] went off and I (. . .) was then taken into the recovery area and I must say <u>that</u> to me (⋆) *that* was horrible because you're just lying there, your baby's taken away from you, and now you're lying there as if, "Okay well, *I'm* the one who produced this baby" and now (⋆) everybody's ^^running about^^ (laughs) (. . .) it's like you're there and going, "Fine, all right, is this it then?" (both laugh) so it was horrible.

Rachelle: It's a bit of a let-down . . .

Carrie: *Ja*, I felt very, <u>ja</u>, that's the exact way I felt, very let down.

                                                                        (White, middle-class)

While some women represented caesarean section as generally just something "that had to happen to get a baby" (Janine), many also wanted the birth experience to be respected and celebrated as a meaningful life event. Several women spoke about being disturbed by the attitudes of medical doctors and staff, who seemed to treat the procedure as, "like another day at the office (laughs) you know it's not a big deal" (Sara) and "an everyday occurrence" (Carrie). While women repeatedly positioned the caesarean as 'no big deal' and, following a medical script, as a mechanical procedure, they also hinted that they longed for it to be treated as something more profound and significant.

Sara: I think the anaesthetist and Mark [husband] were chatting about golf or rugby at some point and I was like, "**Please**, this is an important moment, can we talk about this some other time?" (both laugh) like talking about rugby and they're busy taking my child out (R laughs) so, just pay <u>attention</u> all of you (both laugh).

                                                                        (White, upper class)

Carrie was similarly annoyed that the medical specialists at her birth were, "just chatting away" about "every other thing ^^except what's happening^^." While the body of the woman having a caesarean is the site of copious amounts of (objectified) clinical attention, she is often not treated as a full and whole human person who is undergoing a significant and profound life event (i.e. becoming a mother and giving life) in addition to medical surgery. The distinctiveness of caesarean section as both an everyday and routine surgical procedure *and* as a special profound moment *of birth* needs be recognized and respected by health care professionals.

Violent relations

In addition to forms of 'gentle violence,' modes of embodied oppression and structural disrespect, some women in public sector services were also subject to more overt forms of relational violence. Women thus spoke about the verbal aggression and rough physical treatment they experienced, particularly in MOU settings. Instead of feeling connection, warmth, encouragement and affirmation from their caregivers, some women spoke of being shouted at, bullied, verbally abused, treated rudely and physically mistreated. This created an affective and relational ensemble characterized by negative emotions in which women 'felt bad,' scared and upset. For example:

Cynthia: There was just, she [nurse] wasn't rude but the ways she *talked* was now, was **rude** (R: okay) she doesn't know how to talk, it made me feel very bad.

(Black, low-income, MOU birth)

Rachelle: How would you have liked her [nurse] to have been?

Fadwah: More supportive (★) in the way she spoke to me also (★) like I had struggles with my, with pushing and she could've at least just (★) encouraged me and say something like "It's almost" when it's out you know "It's over" and no, she wasn't, she was rather um (★★) she said, um, "This child is playing with me" (cross voice) "I don't have time for children who play" (cross voice) something like that (R: hmm) and while I was struggling she was walking around and doing her stuff.

(Black, low-income, MOU birth)

These exchanges are narrated as hostile encounters. In the birth assemblages reenacted in these extracts, there is a sense of relational disconnection, lack of basic humane engagement or care and hostility (anger and impatience). In such encounters, women do not feel 'cared for' or 'looked after' but rather receive underlying messages that they are unworthy of care and respect. In addition to being subject to verbal hostilities and affective violence, some women also narrated being physically mistreated. For example, Kuhle spoke about being stitched after birth because of a perineal tear and receiving no anaesthetic during suturing.

Kuhle: Then they came back to stitch me and they they (inaudible) behind the door, like they close the door, they just *uuh* stitch one stitch and then they go to (★) gossip there, then they come back, so when I feel the pain I said #

Rachelle: This is afterwards?

Kuhle: **No, while they are stitching me** because I feel the pain, because (★) **when** they start stitching, I feel the pain and then I say, "Can you give me an injection because I feel the pain," they said, "What do you know because you are not a sister!" *sooo*, it was hard.

(Black, low-income, MOU birth)

This is a form of physical abuse (see Kitzinger, 1992; D'Oliviera, Diniz & Schraibe, 2002). Pain and suffering are inflicted on Kuhle for no good reason. When she exercises agency and asks for a pain injection, she is nullified and subject to a violent exchange—the nurse thus asserts her expert role and reminds Kuhle that she is an ignorant, unknowing and unimportant non-entity. Kuhle is silenced and her bodily experience of pain is denied and dismissed. Even after articulating pain, she is forced to endure suturing with no pain relief. Other women also spoke of being subject to rough physical treatment.

Madiha: I struggled *a lot*. The baby's sugar was *low* and then I had to every time breastfeed *and the child doesn't want to* (. . .) and then they scold me, "Come mommy, come mommy, the child's sugar is low, come, come, come, give the child, give the child" {and so} They didn't **help** you with the (*) to, to latch the child (*) they *vuuh*, that other sister comes in, she ***grrrrgggrrrggghhh***, she <u>pushes</u> that teat *soooo*, the milk <u>shoots out</u>, pushes your {*breasts sore man*}.

(Black, low-income, public hospital birth)

In this exchange, Madiha is depersonalized and treated as a body-object that is simply there to "give the child, give the child" milk. There is no relationship or empathic connection between nurse and mother in this narrated encounter. Instead, Madiha is reprimanded and objectified. Nurses did not talk to her and try to *help* her with latching difficulties but instead treated her as the problem. As a result, she is treated roughly and her body becomes open to forceful and painful manipulations, i.e. "she <u>pushes</u> that teat *soooo* (. . .) pushes your {*breasts sore man*}." In these exchanges it is clear that physical violence and relational violence work in tandem. Moreover, I would argue that it is the subtler forms of invisible, structural and 'gentle' violence present in public sector clinics (denial of personhood, dignity violations, stigmatization) that enable and produce incidents involving more blatant forms of physical and relational violence.

Summary

This chapter explored the violations produced and enacted in birth narratives. In order to move away from analyses that focus on interpersonal modes of birth violence and that enact static victim and perpetrator positions, I focused predominantly on the hidden or invisible forms of violence that were emergent in birth narratives. These forms of violence are slippery, mercurial and evasive, to the point where we are at times left wondering whether 'violence' really occurred or who the 'perpetrator' is/was. Following Žižek (2008), it is these normalized and invisible violences that enable and facilitate the eruptions of direct physical violence and that therefore must be further problematized, exposed and resisted. Often overlooked as 'normal,' the everyday violations of symbolic or 'gentle violence' are sticky and insidious. There often is no clear 'perpetrator.' Instead, there are subjective enactments of powerlessness, loss of agency, obedience and compliance rather than overt force or domination. As a result, symbolic violence does not necessarily leave visceral traces of violence on the flesh. However, as I showed in this chapter, hidden and normalized violences have powerful *affective* consequences, generating compressed and muted subjects, feelings of shame, dehumanization and nullification, and constricted and diminished embodied selves. Operating via insidious and invisible modes of domination, these forms of violence also reiterate normative relations of class, race and gender power.

In relation to labor/birth, this chapter showed that gentle violence, embedded in the norms, sociomaterial and affective flows of assemblages, worked to *generate* passive subjectivities, constricted forms of agency and docile bodies, particularly in public sector contexts. Some women accepted positions of passivity as 'normal' given their marginalized social position/s. Other women reflexively enacted passivity and docility as a strategy to ensure care and avoid mistreatment. The affective threat of violence and neglect was thus often enough to oppress and constrain women during labor/birth. In private sector settings, compliance and obedience was produced as the emergent effect of assemblages in which technoscience, experts, risk discourses, machines and authority relations worked intra-actively to disable women's agency. I also traced the multiple modalities of 'embodied oppression' that materialized in women's stories and argued that heterogeneous forms of power (i.e. biomedical, racialized patriarchy, class) intra-act to enact embodied oppression during labor/birth as everyday and 'normal' within particular birth assemblages. Embodied oppression emerged via multiple modalities of violation, including: interpersonal and technological constraints on embodied agency, violations of dignity and privacy through exposure/s of self and body, shaming, structural disrespect and the denial of embodied personhood. Embodied oppressions were the intra-active effects of colliding forms of power operative in birth assemblages. Biomedical ontologies that enact laboring/birthing bodies as *Körper*—depersonalized, blank body-objects that are separable from the vitalized desiring, needing and feeling energies of embodied selves, functioned as powerful frames enabling a variety of embodied oppressions. These biomedical frames intra-acted with racialized patriarchy and class relations to construct black and poor women's bodies as unworthy of dignity, respect and privacy. Often dignity violations were the effects of structural disrespect and were not traceable to the acts of individual perpetrators. The organization of norms, practices, objects and sociomaterial relations in assemblages were thus structured in/through a broader societal disrespect for birth and the bodies of poor, black women and their infants.

6

RESISTANT BODIES

In the previous three chapters, I explored how normative power relations were intimately interwoven with/in women's choices, expectations, experiences and narratives of birth. In this chapter, I look at the other side of power, namely resistance, subterfuge, countering and subversion. I explore the ways birth narratives leak, counter, exceed, speak back and avoid easy categorization. In efforts to trace how birth narratives themselves function as fluid and emergent assemblages comprised of multiple voices, sociomaterialities and affective layers, I adopt a creative analytic approach, fusing dialogical modes of narrative analysis (Frank, 2010) with poetic representational devices (Gilligan et al., 2003). The aim is to demonstrate the ways in which birth stories cannot be neatly fixed into categories or reduced to single interpretations. Following Frank (2010), I hope to open the reader to the complexity of birth stories as multivocal and contradictory processes of performance, becoming and enactment. There were no singular stories of birth and each voice is "the site of multiple voices" (Frank, 2005, p. 972). While previous chapters explored 'clockwork bodies,' 'risky bodies' and 'violated bodies' as distinctive and coherent narrative threads, narrative 'reality' was a far messier hodgepodge. Women's birth stories were fundamentally multivocal, containing jostling master narratives, heterogenous threads and storylines and a contradictory plurality of voices. Storytelling is a dialogical and sociomaterial process involving dialectical interplay between cultural frames, dominant discourses and fleshy, corpomaterial experience (Ochs & Capps, 1996). As a result of this dynamic and overdetermined multivocality, there are always fugitive spaces available for countering, resistance and push back. Importantly, the listener and the analyst are also part of the dialogical storytelling process. Meanings are not just 'there,' static and waiting to be 'written up'—the listener, analyst and theory methods are intra-acting parts of the research mangle or assemblage. As a result, the kinds of stories told in analysis and research are themselves lively enactments of method, theory and products of affective, corpomaterial flows between tellers, listeners, analysts and readers.

Most conventional modes of qualitative analysis are concerned with categorization and the production of neat, coherent and tidy 'themes.' This means that fledgling and inchoate "moments of strangled articulation, resistance and narrative insight" (Chadwick, 2014, p. 48) are in danger of remaining marginalized and unheard. Subversive and countering voices do not usually emerge fully formed or coherent but often materialize in/through research assemblages as 'moments of excess' (Chadwick, 2014), 'rough spots' (McKendy, 2006) or in/through data that 'glows' (see MacLure, 2013). As MacLure (2013) points out, the analysis of qualitative 'data' is itself a fleshy, entangled and affective process in which analysts are often emotionally and viscerally affected by stories, accounts and tellings that carry the traces of bodily energies, sufferings, joys and the vital pulsing of life. If we want to hear, trace and vitalize 'moments of excess' in narratives, we need to open ourselves to contradictions, incoherence and the embodied and affective power of telling and listening. Moments of narrative excess do not conform to univocal interpretations and are irreducible to categorization. They are often moments in which coherent interpretation stutters, falters and fails. Importantly, excessive moments are often *fleshy eruptions*, in which bodies make their way forcefully into telling—i.e. through laughing, babbling, mumbling, lipsmacking, sighing and crying. They are moments in which the semiotic and corpomaterial aspects of language are vitalized or 'glow' (MacLure, 2013), signaling the possibility of alternative meanings, subterranean resistances or interpretive discontinuities. Unfortunately, it is these radical moments of alterity and corpomaterial disruption that are often regarded as analytic 'debris' (see McKendy, 2006), inconveniences and irrelevant nonsense that needs to be pruned out of transcriptions and analysis. This chapter focuses on 'moments of excess' in birth stories, showing how speaking back and countering often materialized in/through the fleshy, telling body. Narrative resistance was thoroughly embodied, spoken through the suffering, joyful and resistant body. While some forms of resistance emerged 'between the lines,' countering normative discourses via fleshy eruptions, alternative storylines and the production of uncontainable meaning/s, others emerged boldly as efforts to 'push back' against injustice and violation. Interestingly, low-income women enacted the strongest forms of reflexive resistance when they 'spoke back' against mistreatment and inhumane care in public sector services.

Previous chapters showed that medical 'master narratives' (see Nelson, 2001), in the form of clockwork narratives and biomedical risk discourse, framed and dominated women's accounts of birth. Medical frames were, however, always diffracted through race, socioeconomic and gender dynamics and materialized differently within particular assemblages. However, even in the talk of privileged women planning homebirths and low-income women in low-tech maternity settings, telling stories about birth did not seem possible without drawing on biomedical vocabularies (Chadwick, 2009; Kornelsen, 2005). Similarly to Miller (2009, p. 71), women's tellings showed that, "this dominant discourse . . . seeps into women's experiences and stories." Sociomaterial modes of power thus circulated within women's stories as dominant voices, scripts, expectations and corpomaterial relations of violation.

At the same time, however, women's stories also leaked in other directions, enacting modes of resistance, excess, subversion and countering. In this chapter, I trace these moments and articulations of excess and resistance to normative modes of framing birth (and birthing bodies). While medical master narratives and ontological frames continued to be key interpretive frameworks shaping birth stories, in this chapter I trace the subterranean (and sometimes bold) ways women subverted master narratives and found ways of voicing, performing and enacting resistance in/through their birth narratives.

Comic subversive tellings

> The meanings behind laughter reveal both the cracks in the system and the masked or more subtle ways that power is challenged.
>
> *(Goldstein, 2003, p. 5)*

According to Pollock (1999), most birth stories revolve around biomedical complications, danger and 'trouble' with medical experts and interventions often functioning as the active agents of the birth drama. Disaster is often only just averted, with medical technology, interventions and experts saving the day and functioning as narrative 'heroes.' In most conventional birth stories, the birthing woman thus does not feature as the central agent or heroine of labor/birth. Birth is often represented as an ordeal. According to Cosslett (1994, p. 114), everyday birth narratives are often 'horror stories' that emphasize the "pain and drama" of labor/birth. According to narrative analysts, compelling or good stories usually revolve around an unexpected event, complication or 'trouble' (Bruner, 1987; Ochs & Capps, 1996). As a result, I was at first bemused and puzzled by birth stories that seemed to be characterized by a *lack* of narrative 'trouble.' Later I realized that it was their performance of birth as 'trouble-free' that was key to their status as counterstories. Humor, comedy, laughter and funniness pervaded these stories as vitalizing forces; as a result, I named them 'comic subversive' narratives.

The drama of comic subversive narratives did not revolve around biomedical complications. Furthermore, the central agent was the birthing woman and not medical technology or experts. Comic subversive narratives were most prominent among women who planned and experienced birth at home. However, some low-income women giving birth in public sector settings also used a comic subversive style of storytelling. These narratives countered hegemonic medical scripts in which the birthing woman is a passive character in the birth drama. Humor, comedy and laughter characterized this mode of telling and functioned as key moments of uncontainable 'excess' within stories. According to Goldstein (2003, p. 5), humor can reveal points of discontent and "cracks in the system." It is potentially a 'fugitive' form of resistance and is analytically important because it "reveals ambiguity, contradiction, paradox and inconsistency while encouraging multiple interpretations" (p. 6). In the most optimistic sense, humor can be read as a form of 'counter-theatre' in which the marginalized act out subterranean forms of absurdity and defiance (Goldstein, 2003). At the very least, humor can point to ruptures and discontinuities in narratives that can signal moments of subversion or processes of counternarrative (Chadwick, 2014).

Birth was not represented as a harrowing 'ordeal' in comic subversive stories but as fun and often enjoyable. In the context of hegemonic biomedical risk discourses, and the pervasiveness of birth storytelling that emphasizes complications, pain and the 'horrors' of birth, this mode of storytelling disrupts sociocultural norms. Told in a comic vein, comic subversive tellings were filled with 'funny little stories' and characterized by abundant laughing and giggling. The source of the humor was often the subversive quality of the stories themselves as they managed to overturn and disrupt many cultural assumptions about how birth should proceed (and be narrated). Instead of being an ordeal or a horror story, homebirth was referred to, for example, as "a party" (Maggie) or "a breeze" (Suzette). Medicalized modes of birth were disrupted by stories that represented birth as a time of fun, everyday normality and ease. Particularly in the middle-class context of the South African private sector, which is saturated by grueling stories of birth in which multiple complications and caesarean sections have become the norm (see Keeton, 2010), middle-class women are expected to tell birth stories filled with 'things going wrong' and a plethora of technological interventions (Humphreys, 1998).

Birth heroines and funny little stories

In comic subversive narratives, birthing women emerged as the true heroines of birth. For example, Maggie told the story of her first homebirth (after two previous private hospital births), in a comic vein in which birth was reproduced as a normal, everyday, social event—in her words: "like a party." The astounding 'normalcy' of the scenes in her narrative work, in a comic fashion, to disrupt medical horror stories of birth. For example:

Maggie: My waters had broken and I was, by the time she [assistant midwife] arrived here, and once he [baby] was out, "Hi Tina!" (R laughs) and she said, "It's nice to meet you Maggie, I recognize you from X, you used to work there?" I said, "Yes" and she goes, "Well done my girl, you've do(ne) it, you've been amazing." I said, "Thank you, I'm hungry now, ↑can I have MacDonald's?"↑ (R laughing) ^^I was *starving* already^^ (both laughing) Mark's [partner] mom had made sandwiches (. . .) you know what the amazing thing was? (R: yes?) He was born **here** [home], I got up within 10 minutes, they helped me to bed, and I lay with him and Mark in the bed, they ran a bath and the two of us bathed together, and within 45 minutes my kids were here and I was sitting outside having a cup of tea and a sandwich, the neighbors had popped in already, the house was *full* of people, it was like a party (R: oh wonderful) I didn't feel like I had just been through (*) having a baby. And by the time I, like I was in the bath, they cleaned everything up, when I came through everything was cleaned up, I walked around and I picked up a few towels and packed away and they said, "Relax," I said, "I'm fine, I don't feel like I just had a baby," ^^"I'm just hungry, can someone make me another sandwich please?^^ (laughs).

(White, planned homebirth)

In this narrative extract, ordinary events such as asking for a 'MacDonald's' or a sandwich become funny and comic, because the requests are coming from a woman who has just (minutes before) *given birth*. Commonsense storylines of birth assume that women should, at this stage, be acting like 'patients' who have just been through a medical ordeal. Women are not supposed to sit up promptly after giving birth, say they are 'starving' and demand food. In Maggie's story, the immediate aftermath of birth does not involve machines, pain, hospital equipment, wound repair, sterilizing treatments, the surveillance of medical experts or sequestration. Instead, the post-birth scene is a social and domestic scene filled with friends, family, celebration, sandwiches and tea, and normal household activities. Maggie contrasted this homebirth with a previous private hospital birth experience. She described disappointment and a sense of isolation as her dominant affective responses to giving birth in a (private) hospital.

Maggie: I felt disappointed because they, they take your baby away, well as soon as you give birth in hospital, you hold them for a few minutes and then they take it away to be weighed and cleaned and then (. . .) while they're doing all the tests and they're dressing your baby and all that kind of stuff, and they bring it to you all dressed and you're actually, you're sitting there like *nah-nah-nah-nah-nah*, okay I've had, I've done, I've just done something exciting—now what was it? (R laughs) and you're waiting for, you're waiting for this child and you're just sitting all by yourself (★) and your husband is either with you or he's with the baby being bathed and cleaned and being made <u>presentable</u> for you, you know, you don't see your baby covered in all the vernix and all that kind of stuff, it gets cleaned up, your baby gets brought to you smelling like a Johnson's ad.

Underlined by a sense of separation between mother and baby, rituals of purification and measurement, Maggie is alienated from her newborn baby in the standard medical script. In contrast, immediately after giving birth at home, Maggie and her newborn had a bath together, which she describes as "the most *normal* thing to do." Throughout her telling of post-birth scenes at home she constantly reiterates that, "I didn't feel like I just had a baby." What she means here is that she didn't feel like a woman who has just given birth is expected to feel within medicalized birth assemblages and according to normative medical scripts of birth—i.e. exhausted, out-of-it and the survivor of a harrowing medical 'ordeal.' The story thus subverts hegemonic cultural recipes for telling birth narratives and it is subversion that produces its humorous effects. The comic subversive narrative is humorous and countering in relation to other (predominantly medical) narrative templates that inscribe what is 'normal' in relation to birth.

Maggie told her birth story as a series of comic sub-plots, all of which worked ultimately to counter master narratives of birth as a medical event, potentially traumatic, horrifying and prone to malfunction and complications. For example, consider the following 'funny little story':

Maggie: I was walking down the street and the neighbors would say, "When are you having your baby?" I said, "Now"—"What do you mean—<u>now</u>?" I said, "I'm in labor," "Then go inside." I said, "No" (both laugh), I said, "I like these lamp-posts, I like these little, it's my holding-on stations" cause I've been living here for 12 years (R: okay) so I know, I know most of the neighbors, and it was divine, it was, they were all, "We're looking forward to seeing the balloons outside"—we were going to put balloons outside to show whether it was a boy or a girl, so the neighbors were all like, the whole street was like (R: waiting?) sitting . . . one neighbor came out at about half past one, my parents had just arrived, she said, "You're having this baby?" I was standing behind the car, she couldn't see me, I said, "I've **had** it," she goes, "What do you mean you've had it?" I said, "Look, it's gone," she says, "When did you have it?" I said, "An hour and a half ago," she goes "*Oh my god*! And she runs inside (R laughs) and she runs across the road and she gives me this present and she goes, "But you don't *look* like you've just had a baby," I said, "I don't *feel* like I've just had a baby."

The narrative 'trouble' driving Maggie's birth story is the fact that there were no problems, complications or difficulties. Birth is experienced as smooth and easy and takes place without fuss. Birth is also not sequestrated from everyday life and takes place within a social and community environment. Maggie does not stay hidden inside her house but ventures around the neighborhood while in labor, boldly claiming public space. As a result, there is some consternation from her neighbors as she materially enacts the disruption of social norms. The unexpected and disruptive impact of 'trouble-free' homebirth on the general public is comically demonstrated by the incredulous and funny reactions of Maggie's neighbors, who are characterized as astounded and shocked by their collision with a birth story that defies all accepted cultural norms and expectations. Maggie's narrative is multivocal, involving a complex weave of voices including the assumed medical master narrative (birth is a risky ordeal that should take place in a hospital), Maggie's fuss-free and thus subversive homebirth, and a comical audience of incredulous neighbors.

In a similar vein, Suzette described her homebirth as "a breeze" and described birth as an unremarkable and everyday part of life. After bathing with the baby after birth, she "put normal clothing on and went for a walk the afternoon and friends came over." Like Maggie, her birth narrative was comprised of 'funny little stories' that typically involved 'gob-smacked' neighbors. For example, she describes one of the neighbors as completely dumbfounded by her incredibly quick birth experience, which lasted less than two hours.

Suzette: I phoned the morning, at quarter to eight, I phoned the neighbor cause I know she's going to the early service at church (R: yes) and I asked her can my parents maybe go with her and she said no, she's not going um today cause her daughter's visiting or whatever, and so my parents went on their own, but then she decided she wants to go to the second service at ten and when she left for the second service, the pink balloons were hanging in front of the gate (R laughs) and she said she's sitting through the whole service, thinking, "Why do we put balloons up?" ^^because at eight I didn't say anything!^^

(White, planned homebirth)

Several other homebirthers (e.g. Jolene, Jane, Erin, Joni and Jeannie) told birth in a similar dashing and comic subversive style in which the ease and everyday 'normality' of the birth event functioned as the key mode of narrative 'trouble.' However, it was not only middle-class women who had homebirths that told birth as a comic subversive narrative. Positive experiences of giving birth in public sector settings were also sometimes told via this narrative type. For example, similarly to the privileged, middle-class participants above, Sarayda told her birth narrative (which took place in a public hospital) via comic sub-plots and 'funny little stories' in which she starred as the heroine.

Sarayda: I walked *a lot* everyday, so all of that helped to give me an easy birth, so that was why it was just 45 minutes! (R: Wow!) When I, when I phoned my daughter back, cause they thought I'm gonna be there [public hospital] for a day and a night and that, and I got up and I had my child in the trolley and I pushed her to the phone and I was on the phone—*they just got home*—and I said (loud laughing) (R: I've already had the baby!) my daughter answered and I said, "Yes, it's mommy here and she said, "Why are you on the phone? Why aren't you laying down? Aren't you in pain?" (Agitated voice), She said, "I don't know what's wrong with this woman?" I said, "Listen to me, I want to tell you something—I gave birth already," she said, "OH NO ^^there's something definitely wrong!^^ (both laugh) she said to Simon [daughter's boyfriend] "My mommy had a baby already!" And I said, "Its a girl" . . . "And it's a girl! The baby's there!—And we have to go back now!"

(Black, low-income, public hospital birth)

In a similar style to the comic subversive narratives told by Maggie and Suzette, Sarayda's story delights in conveying how shocked and astounded those around her were by her easy and trouble-free birth experience. In the extract, Sarayda's relatives are cast as the dumbstruck audience that are left reeling and disbelieving when confronted with a birth story that clashes with cultural expectations that birth should take a long time, be painful and in which birthing women should be "laying down" and behaving like patients. Sarayda's daughter is depicted as constantly voicing the suspicion that something is wrong with her mother because she is not conforming to expectations about how a woman-in-labor should behave—i.e. "what's wrong with this woman?"

Importantly, while representing birth as normal and uncomplicated, comic subversive narratives also reproduced birthing women as the central and active agents of the birth event. There was often a strong and distinctive sense of embodied agency and fleshy knowing accompanying these stories. Women stressed contentment and satisfaction with their birth experiences. Jane (white, planned homebirth) described her birth as "thrilling," Maggie (white, planned homebirth) said that birth was, "one of the best experiences I've ever had," Charné (black, public hospital birth) said that, "it was fun, it was nice" and according to Bronwyn, birth was "^^the best time of my life^^" (Black, public hospital birth). Women also expressed a sense of pride in how they had managed the bodily birthing process. For example:

Sarayda: Seriously, it was a nice experience, it was really, and when we got to the hospital they [relatives] said they must bring me a wheelchair, they shouted to the nurses they must bring me a wheelchair, I said, "I don't want a wheelchair," I walk myself in there and then the nurses in the labor ward, um, my daughter's boyfriend, then he said, "The lady's in-labor—can you please see to her?" And then the nurses look at him and they say "Sir, but she's fine—this lady looks quite fine to us (R laughs) you don't have to shout like that cause she is not shouting, she's okay—so that experience for me was beautiful, I really *experienced* everything because of the, my water that broke and my contractions coming like that, I knew exactly how to do it—for myself, without anybody telling me.

(Black, low-income, public hospital birth)

This extract beams and brims with bodily pleasure and contentment. There is also a strong sense of embodied agency, knowing and personal capacity reproduced here—as Sarayda says, "I knew exactly how to do it—for myself, without anybody telling me." Maggie also spoke about feeling proud and 'warm' about her comic subversive birth.

Maggie: When I look at the benefits, and that sense of, that self of self, that I've actually done it, I've, I've, I did it for me (. . .) it's, it just makes you **feel** (*) a whole lot of different things, it's like a "I did it" kind of proud thing as opposed to . . . it's a *warm* feeling cause I, I, it was one of the best experiences I've ever had.

(White, planned homebirth)

While birth was foregrounded as a *normal event* in the comic subversive narrative, women did not necessarily minimize or mute the pain of the labor/birth experience. Instead, they reframed pain as something that was manageable and expected; according to Suzette, "I *know* it's gonna be heavy and I *know* it's gonna be sore, so when it arrived I knew it's here and I mean I enjoyed it (both laugh)." Coping well with pain and feelings of satisfaction/pleasure were thus associated with being able to enact active forms of embodied agency during labor/birth.

While embodied agency and a sense of ownership of the birth experience were often partners and products of comic subversive tellings, it is important to note that these tellings were embedded in affirming, caring and supportive connections with others. Relational, sociomaterial and affective economies together with bodily and physiological factors shape the kind/s of embodied agency that women are able to enact during birth. While comic subversive narratives disrupted normative assumptions about birth as predominantly a medical event defined by biomedical risks, complications and best managed by medical experts, they were not free-floating narratives but were enactments of affirming sociomaterial and relational assemblages.

Relational assemblages

Comic subversive stories created performative spaces for presence, resistance and embodied agency during birth tellings, and subverted definitions of birth as a medical event. These stories were, however, also sociomaterial products of birth assemblages characterized by warmth and caring relations. Being able to construct forms of bodily agency during birth was linked to receiving body-to-body support and encouragement from others. In comic subversive narratives, women were almost always tangibly and deeply embedded in a matrix of bodily connections with their caregivers and birth supporters. The potential entanglement of bodies in such assemblages, in which the birthing woman, caregiver, partner and supporters became almost indistinguishable, was powerfully illustrated in some stories. For example:

Lizette: You see it was also going with support hey, I mean if you imagine the scene with Paul [partner] behind me, and I'm standing, and my sister's on, at my left leg and the midwife's at my right leg, and my foot was actually on them, on their laps or legs or something, I dunno, my feet wasn't on the ground cause I kept slipping on the ground for some reason, so they held my feet and then there's, then there's another midwife who's there next to the other midwife, like say in the middle, and I'm standing and then I would, then I would feel the contraction come and then I would go <u>down</u> and I would say, "Okay, it's coming" and then you would just have everybody's energy and everybody's attention like on you and it would be "*Aaahhuuuhh*" and everybody's "*Aaahhuuuhh-ing*" with me (R laughs) and you know, and the midwife says, "Go now, push, push, push, well done—okay, breath out again, breath in and carry on pushing from there" you know and they're all like right <u>there</u>, it's not just, kind of me sitting pushing (R: hmm) like somewhere, everybody's making *a noise* as well so I didn't feel like <u>I</u> was (R: the only one) grunting or anything, like everyone was sort of grunting with me . . .

(White, planned homebirth)

This narrative enactment illustrates the power of affirming, body-to-body connections during labor/birth. Lizette is not isolated or sharply differentiated from others. The scene contrasts dramatically with imagery produced in the stories of other women (see particularly Chapter 5), in which they were regularly constructed as passive, sequestrated patients that were 'observed,' ignored or treated as body-objects to be practiced upon. In the scene from Lizette's story, there is no external observer (everyone present is a participant) and she is not cast as a spectacle or object in any sense. Instead, she is the pulsating center of a supportive and strongly embodied (stroking, massaging, holding, grunting) hub of intermeshed bodies. Lizette becomes a 'body-without-boundaries' entangled with other bodies to the point where her self-contained and individual separateness is questioned; as she says: "I didn't feel like <u>I</u> was grunting or anything."

Sarayda's comic subversive narrative of birth, in which she enacted a strong sense of embodied agency—"I could do everything for myself"—and fleshy pleasure, was also embedded in a caring and supportive (public sector) birth assemblage.

Rachelle: Were they [nurses] with you most of the time?
Sarayda: They were with me ALL the time.
Rachelle: You weren't left alone?
Sarayda: No, all the time, I felt like a <u>celebrity </u>there, the treatment they gave me, it was very, it was very nice the treatment they gave me, checked every time—"Is my pillows okay? How are you feeling?" Checking my pulse and damping my head from the sweat and all of that (*) they were really, they were full-on, they were nice (. . .) they were so like um, they were really part of everything there with me.

(Black, low-income, public hospital)

Sarayda emphasized that caregivers should be active participants in the birth experience. As demonstrated in narratives, the affective environment of birth is critical in enabling capacities, forms of bodily agency and satisfying experiences. Comic subversive stories and resistant storylines were often entangled with/in affirming birth assemblages. Enacting agency, living and coping with the bodily sensations of labor/birth and *feeling* power and presence materialized as the intra-active products of supportive environments and caring others. Women narrated positive birth experiences in which they were agents and heroines, when they were warmly located within a mesh of connectivity and body-to-body support.

While most comic subversive narratives were embedded in warm and affirming relational assemblages, there was one participant who managed to transform a negative affective birthing environment (in the public sector) into a comic story that dramatized the relational encounter/s between nurse/patient as a humorous battle of wills. Rizwana, a young Muslim woman pregnant with her first baby, told a story of giving birth in the local MOU as a comic subversive drama involving a humorous to-and-fro struggle with nurses. While describing birth as partly an experience of distress in which she felt alone and scared, and in which nurses were often angry and harsh with her, Rizwana was also able to draw on a comic subversive genre to reconstruct the birth as a humorous drama filled with funny micro-stories, humor, laughter and fleshy energies. In her story, she constructs her self as the active protagonist (or heroine) constantly engaged in small acts of resistance and as active in 'speaking back' in the face of efforts to control and punish her during labor/birth. As a result, in her story, birth was reproduced as a relational, resistant and comic dance between 'powerful' authorities (i.e. the nurses) that tried to exert control via domination, and the birthing woman, who constantly 'pushed back' at efforts to suppress by demanding, countering and exerting resistance and agency. For example:

Rizwana: And then I walked up and down because they take their own time (laughs), walked up and down and then they said "No, don't walk, you must lie down" then I said, "No sister, the pain is sore," "No, did you think having a baby *is nice*?" (Smacks lips) I said, "No sister I can't say that but I want to walk," they say "No, lie down" (both laughing) And I showed them I am **very stubborn**, showed them I walk, they got *angry*, then I lay down and then I screamed "*Sister!*" and she said, "Yes man we are busy!" "Sister, the pains sister!" "No man we are busy now" (R laughs) I think okay ^^ they are busy! ^^ (R laughs) I can walk again now (R laughing), when they saw me up again then they scolded, then the ***other*** sister said to the (★) other sister "Leave her alone—let her walk around" (★) "But if she is already complaining so much how is she going to be when she has to push? I said, "^^Don't worry sister about how I am going to complain when I push^^ (R laughs) ^^the pains—just help me! ^^

(Black, low-income, MOU birth)

Rizwana's entire birth story continued in this vein, telling labor and birth as a series of lively, relational skirmishes with nurses. Instead of being cowered and 'muted' by the behavior of nurses, Rizwana (narratively at least) found ways of resisting, fighting back and exerting forms of agency. The relational nature of power is beautifully illustrated in this comic subversive narrative. In her story, mistreatment is transformed into comedy and she manages to enact reflexive forms of resistance in which she stars as the heroine and central agent of the birth drama. At the same time, it is important to note that her story was not singular or seamlessly resistant; Rizwana told her birth experience as a dialogical weave between a humorous comic subversive drama and a 'narrative of distress' in which she articulated her loneliness, fear and anxiety during labor/birth.

Fleshy and excessive tellings

> It is only 'audience' point of view narratives that are able to give single and simple accounts of childbirth: experienced from the centre, that 'centre' becomes diffuse, multiple, fractured.
>
> (Cosslett, 1994, p. 118)

While most women framed their birth stories within biomedical vocabularies, risk discourses and clockwork scripts, there was often *another kind of story* that rode alongside and against dominant narratives. This was not a coherent or linear narrative but a strongly embodied telling that told the visceral, pulsating and psychofleshy experience of labor/birth. Bodily eruptions and moments of fleshy excess were key characteristics of these tellings. As a result, births were told in a lively style and often at a dizzying pace, overflowing with an abundance of animated words, fleshy energies, pitch fluctuations, loud vocalizations and affective intensities of joy and pleasure or suffering, chaos and distress. These fleshy tellings contrasted starkly with clockwork and passive narratives in which labor/birth were told via technical, formulaic language and with little sense of body, flesh, lived experience or *joie de vivre*. Working as a semiotic force, fleshy tellings disrupted the coherence and linear lines of medical and clockwork narratives, working to resist and subvert normativity, univocality and single interpretations of birth.

Given that these were often subterranean articulations, how did I come to recognize or hear fleshy and excessive tellings? Early on in the analysis process, when I was listening to audio-recordings of interviews, I began to *feel* that fleshy bodies were tangible presences in birth stories, crackling in/through the recordings and constantly interrupting my efforts to herd meaning into patterns, coherence and neatly packaged interpretations. I did not know what to do with these bodies or how to think about them. Searching for a way of making sense, I wrote in my research journal at the time:

> Voices are alive. Meaning crackles in-between words: in breaths, rhythms, a myriad of laughters, pauses, spaces in-between, rising and lowering pitch, snapping fingers and guttural sounds (that are difficult to convert into conventional alphabetic letters). The dance between the interviewee and myself—my interruptions, my nervous laughter, my awkwardness—hanging—suspended in questions that trail off . . .

Early on in analysis I was thus attuned to the radical inseparability of bodies and language and intuitively sensed that there is, "something wild in language: something that exceeds propositional meaning and resists the laws of representation"

(MacLure, 2013, p. 658). I was viscerally affected by the 'data'; it made me feel things. The theoretical work of Julia Kristeva (see Chapter 1) later helped me to think about the complex entanglements between bodies, speech, feelings, language and 'data.' New materialist approaches also provide ways of thinking about 'data analysis' that embrace the vitality of data itself and acknowledge its material and affective agency (see MacLure, 2013). As a result, data can 'glow' and affect us (MacLure, 2013) evoking sensations and visceral feelings in researchers/ analysts. Rather than muting or managing the uncontainable eruptions and affective forces of fleshy bodies in language, we need to stay with them and their trouble (Haraway, 2016) and trace their potentialities for disruption, alternative interpretations and countering.

Women told two kinds of fleshy counterstories, one that produced pleasure and joy and another that told corpomaterial experiences of trauma and distress. The key feature of fleshy counterstories was that they were told from the fleshy onto- logical perspective of birthing women and thus produced embodied stories spoken performatively from the laboring/birthing body. Similarly to Frank's (1995) chaos narrative, these were not fully-fledged narratives with clear temporal ordering but rather 'ways of telling' that countered master narratives of birth characterized by out- sider, observer or audience perspectives of birth (i.e. biomedical and phallocentric). Fleshy tellings of labor/birth were similar to what Frank (1995) refers to as 'chaos narratives' but also different in significant ways. According to Frank's (1995) analysis of illness narratives, chaos narratives represented the "most embodied form of story" (p. 101) fixated on an "incessant present" (p. 99) marked by suffering, bottomless despair, pain and loss of control. The chaotic body was told as isolated and unable to find recognition or support. Frank (1995) identifies a particular style of telling, characterized by hurried and repeated references to 'and then . . . and then . . . and then,' as an identifying feature of chaos narratives. In these narratives, the story- teller is overwhelmed by a chaos that cannot be adequately put into words. "In the most hurried 'and then' telling, chaos is the ultimate muteness that forces language to go faster and faster, trying to catch the suffering in words" (Frank, 1995, p. 102). While women's 'fleshy ways of telling' were also often marked by the 'and then . . . and then . . . and then' speech style and were thoroughly embodied stories, they often worked to inscribe *pleasure, bodily engagement and agency* rather than despair and loss of meaning. The 'and then' style of telling occurred in both fleshy tellings of pleasure and distress but differed in terms of what kinds of bodily and affective energies and modes of agency were produced. Fleshy tellings of distress enacted a loss of agency, a sense of being overwhelmed and traced wounds of loss, trauma and pain. Fleshy tellings of pleasure produced embodied agency, positive energies and a sense of joy, exuberance, power and connection.

Telling fleshy pleasure

Comic subversive narratives, as explored in the previous section, were dialogically entangled with other storylines and often rode alongside fleshy modes of telling that seeped and swirled with bodily pleasure/s. While 'the body' was hardly ever mentioned in these fleshy tellings, birth was itself told as a pleasurable form of body talk in which the movements, visceral sensations and embodied emotions of the birthing woman became the center of a living and moving story.

Erin: I started writing an email because there, there was something I'd, I'd left <u>undone</u>, sort of a work-related thing (. . .) and um, and then (★) the, the contractions started getting a little bit stronger and I was, I was sort of rocking backwards and forwards on this bouncy ball (. . .) so I went and wrote my email quickly (★) and in-between sort of *rocked* between contractions and stuff and then I sent it and she [midwife] said, "Okay, let's do it" [break waters] so she um, broke my waters (★) and there must have been about two litres of fluid that came out (R: Gee!) it was *amazing*, it just came and came and came, **the bed was wet** and (giggles) (R: Oh my goodness!) towels were *soaked* (R laughs) and then the contractions got quite (★) intense, quick, quick after that, so um, and with, with Amy [first baby] all I wanted to do through the contractions was just lie down and chill (R: hmm) and with this little one I wanted to, <u>to rock</u> (. . .) um I just, I walked around, put some music on and I walked around the bedroom and every time a contraction came, I'd sort of **grab** Luke [husband] and rock and then, and that went on for a while, and the contractions kind of got more and more intense, um and Dolores [midwife] <u>ran a bath</u> and said, "Anytime you want to, get in the bath" so I sort of left that until I ***knew*** I <u>really</u> needed to get in the bath and um (. . .) um (★) I think it was all very <u>unstressful</u> . . .

(White, planned homebirth)

In this extract, Erin tells her birth story by centering herself as a moving, active, desiring and embodied self. She does not refer to external dilation measurements (centimeters and minutes) or plot her body according to clocktime codes. Instead, the 'I' that is performed in this extract is active, knowing and strongly embodied. This is dramatically illustrated by pulling out the 'I' voice statements within her talk.

I started . . . I'd . . . I'd . . . I was rocking . . . I went . . . I wrote . . . I sent it . . . I wanted . . . I wanted to rock . . . I just . . . I walked . . . I walked . . . I'd grab . . . I sort of . . . I knew . . . I really needed . . . I think . . . I . . . I could . . . I thought . . . I want . . .

As opposed to medical narratives of birth (i.e. clockwork narratives), there is little sense in Erin's story of a separation between 'a body' and 'a mind.' The subject performed in this telling is embodied, flowing and desiring. She moves and acts in accordance with bodily needs, urges and desires. Contractions come and go and get stronger and more intense. Erin focuses on how they *felt* and does not objectify labor according to external interpretive codes. The story moves, breathes and enacts the fleshy bodily experience of labor. Along with this telling comes a sense of bodily pleasure and amazement at the power of the body-in-labor. Erin describes the flow of amniotic fluid as, "*amazing*, it just came and came and came, **the bed was wet** and (giggles) towels were *soaked.*"

Although pleasure-filled fleshy tellings and 'body talk' were most prominent in the accounts of middle-class women who had planned homebirths, they were also evident in the stories of low-income women giving birth in the public sector. For example:

Sarayda: I went for a walk and then when I got home and I went to sit down, my waters broke (R: okay), I never experienced that with the first one, so that was a nice experience for me—feeling that '*buuuuuphhh.*'

Rachelle: A nice experience?

Sarayda: It was a very nice feeling (R: Really?) it was <u>very nice</u> (. . .) so when I sat down and I felt this '<u>guuuuusssh</u>' like this, I actually felt the bubble in my stomach, it opened, it burst and that was <u>so nice</u> (R laughs) and the water *came out*, I'm like "Wow! This is nice!" (R laughs) (. . .) I said, "<u>My water just *burst*</u>! ^^It's *so nice*^^ (R laughs) and then it burst again for a second, I said, "*Wow*—<u>again</u>—^^if you can only know this experience!^^ (both laughing).

(Black, low-income, public hospital birth)

The potentially tactile and sensual pleasures involved in *feeling* the bodily sensations of labor cannot be articulated or spoken within medical or phallocentric narratives of birth. In fleshy tellings, however, there was space for the sensual body to speak back and be re-enacted via storytelling. In the extract above, the embodied telling itself is suffused with uncontainable bodily eruptions as evidenced by the use of sounds such as "*buuuuuphhh*" and "<u>guuuuussh</u>." A sense of fleshy pleasure is reproduced in and through the rhythm, tones and vocalizations of the telling. Sarayda conveys a sense of enlargement, amazement and satisfaction ("that was <u>so nice</u>") at the tactile bodily sensations she experienced during labor. In a similar vein, Mandy narrated the moment of birth itself as intensely tactile, powerful and potentially ecstatic. Her performative telling of this moment is volatile, exuberant and brimming with bodily joy and pleasure.

Mandy: Um and then she [midwife] said, "All right, so now with the third push, you're gonna crown her" and she said, "Otherwise all your pushes are going to be in vain (R: hmm) so just push her and crown her, and then we'll work it from there" and then, I decided, just like that, I'm not going, I'm not going half measures, so I just pushed *incredibly hard* on the third contraction, and then pushed her out (laughs).

Rachelle: Just like that?

Mandy: ^^Yes, and everyone got quite a fright because they weren't expecting it, it's so funny!^^ (. . .) um (*) and then Dolores was going, "Yes, that's right, there she's crowned, OH SHE'S COMING, OH NO, HER HEAD'S OUT, HER HEAD'S OUT (R laughing) OH GOD, YE(s) (laughing) she's her(e) (both laughing) It was so funny (. . .) and then still on all fours hey, I pushed her to me, through my legs, and gave her a little **_kiss_** from her mom.

(White, planned homebirth)

Mandy's telling is subversive on several levels. Against medical models of birth, the birthing woman is inscribed with authority and control and decides "just like that" that she is going to do things for herself and not follow medical instructions. The commonsense, medicalized view that the birthing body is made up of a series of fragmented 'parts'—i.e. uterus, cervix, vagina—which work separately, involuntarily and purely physiologically (without the subjective involvement of the birthing woman) to birth babies (see Sbisà, 1996), is also disrupted. In the extract, Mandy decides to give birth, actively does it and then laughs in the face of the incredulous midwife and other birth supporters. Infusing her talk is also a powerful sense of embodied pleasure, evidenced by laughter, loud vocalizations and lively speech rhythms. As a counter to the biomedicalized birthing body (silenced and objectified), the birthing body is enacted as sensual, powerful, active, joyous and potentially ecstatic.

Fleshy storylines of pleasure were thus suffused with a sense of fun, joy and success and operated in a pleasurable way, eliciting laughter and positive affective energies. According to Pollock (1999), birth stories rarely conclude with "complete satisfaction" (p. 4). In fleshy tellings of birth pleasure, however, stories resonated with a thorough sense of satisfaction and absolute contentment. For example:

Jane: Yes, it was really **good** (R laughs) ^^*in fact I really want, want to have another one now* (R: Really?) *to see if I can do it all over again!*^^ (laughing)

Rachelle: That's fantastic!

Jane: Yes, it was, it was a **good** birth.

(White, planned homebirth)

Jasmine, an extremely impoverished woman living in destitute conditions, invoked a pleasure-filled fleshy narrative when talking about her experience of giving birth at home with no birth attendant. As outlined in earlier chapters, Jasmine 'chose' to birth at home unattended instead of giving birth at the local MOU because she feared stigmatization, public shaming and mistreatment.

Jasmine: I was sitting here [home], I had a jeans on, the pains coming, *I was shouting* SAY TWO OR THREE TIMES and the neighbors, the neighbors are very supportive, the neighbors <u>came</u> and I was sitting there "*Come, come* to the doctor" but they, they do(n't), they don't **<u>understand</u>**—the pain also but the other thing was I don't want to, cause then, *they're gonna skel [scold] me out also* and I was, it's almost like a <u>poops</u> that wants to come out and the <u>poops</u> is, so I started ^^to

poops there^^ but I feel the, I thought it's **the head** or something
^^the poops but I still feel here IN FRONT pressing there^^ still pressing there and they said, "**Come, let's still do it now**" [go to clinic]
every time, "**No, the head's coming out!**," they said "*No, come!*"
(. . .) I was pressing, pressing, I feel just a head, someone was shouting here "THERE'S THE HEAD" the people's coming, everyone
(R laughs) everyone! Everyone ^^it was like a matric ball here outside^^
(both laughing) and I feel *the body* and I'm saying "God help me."

(Black, low-income, unplanned homebirth)

Jasmine tells a powerfully fleshy and multivocal birth story. The fleshy pleasures,
energies and intense corporeality of labor/birth are transfused and reperformed
in her telling. Fleshy re-enactment is achieved via loud vocalizations, the bodily rhythms of the speech, laughter, humor and variations in pitch and emphasis.
Riding alongside the fleshy, pleasure-laden telling are, however, also externalized
voices of interruption, which refer to the need for medical help and intervention.
Her neighbors, who gather around to help and support her during the birth, are
keen to deliver her to the clinic and to "the doctor" as the general consensus in
the community seems to be that birth must happen in a medical setting with health
care professionals. Jasmine has to wrestle not only with the fleshy birth experience
but she also has to struggle to stay out of the maternity clinic and the mistreatment
that she sees as inevitable in this space. She exerts agency and resistance both via
her insistence on birthing outside the (in her view dysfunctional) system and via a
fleshy counterstory of birth, which inscribes her as the living, feeling and pulsating
center of the labor/birth experience.

Jasmine's narrative is also comic subversive as it describes the humorous scene
in which neighbors pile in to be part of the birth drama and excitement—as she
says, "the people's coming, everyone, everyone! Everyone ^^it was like a matric
ball outside^^." Unable to access and afford private birth attendants (i.e. private
midwives) means that Jasmine's 'homebirth' does not run to the same script as
middle-class 'homebirthers.' She is vulnerable to significant risks that middle-class
women planning homebirths easily avoid. At the same time, outside of the stric-
tures of medicalized modes of birth, she is able to flow with and fully experience
the birth without having to deal with mistreatment, rude comments, stigmatization
and dignity violations from public sector health care professionals. As she said later
in the interview:

Rachelle: And the birth –are you glad it happened here?
Jasmine: Yes, ^^I'm very glad^^ (both laugh) ^^I'M VERY GLAD IT
HAPPENED HERE^^ I'm very glad and it was quick also (. . .) you
would have had the pain there also—the, the sisters they would've
walked up and down the whole time, they will <u>ignore</u> you because I
had that experience before (. . .) they will ignore you, it's almost like
"You don't talk the truth, you don't know when the baby is gonna
come" that kind of stuff.

According to Jasmine, giving birth in the MOU is an experience of 'pain.' By 'pain' she means not the physical pain of labor/birth but the emotional pain and suffering caused by mistreatment. In clinic settings, women's embodied knowledge of labor and birth is routinely dismissed and they were made to feel as though they "don't talk the truth." At home Jasmine was able to avoid the denigration of her privileged access to the fleshy sensations of labor/birth and become a 'loud body' (Shabot, 2016) without censure or restriction. While walking a tightrope between a birth experience free of violations, and in her words "life and death" risks due to the lack of any birth attendant or medical care, Jasmine's fleshy telling is multivocal, performing pleasure and excitement with risk and danger hovering and humming alongside. As explored in Chapter 5, low-income women often narrated birth experiences in which their efforts to enact forms of embodied agency and flow with their bodies during labor/birth were met with punishment, forms of violation and embodied oppression/s. As explicated there, medical models of birth (and medical professionals) are potentially challenged and 'troubled' by the subversive and 'loud bodies' engendered by labor and birth (Shabot, 2016). As a result, efforts to 'control,' mute and regulate these noisy bodies materialize in a variety of ways including the use of pharmacological drugs, interventions, policing and surveillance and relational forms of punishment and modes of 'discipline.' Middle-class women giving birth at home were largely protected from these outside interruptions and thus, not surprisingly, were able to enact, perform and tell stories of subversive, fleshy and empowering forms of birthing agency and bodily pleasure.

Fleshy narratives inscribing pleasure were not univocal. Furthermore, pleasure was often paradoxical and incorporated loss of control, pain and struggle. For example, the loss of individualist notions of 'control' often accompanied pleasure-laden, fleshy narratives of birth. As a result, this was not a loss of control that signaled suffering, trauma or distress. Instead, it paradoxically affirmed embodied agency and a sense of bodily achievement. Through complex embodied engagements, women were able to flow with the laboring and birthing body and enact forms of bodily agency. Often paradoxical modes of control were invoked in which women spoke about gaining agency by letting go of ideals of self-contained control. For example:

Lizette: I didn't feel like I was *out* of control, I didn't feel that I was like spinning out of control in *that* way, but I felt that I was in a process, I was on the wave, you know, these waves kept coming and I had entered into that realm and I was there but that, that realm wasn't my doing (. . .) you're not in control of what's happening and you're not in control, but yes, you're, for most of it I was in control as far as I was letting go into the process.

(White, planned homebirth)

Jolene: You have to try and control the pain by giving into it.

(Black, middle-class, homebirth)

Birth is a unique psychofleshy experience in which pain, satisfaction and joy are intertwined in complex and distinctive ways that differ radically from other experiences of bodily pain such as illness or injury. During labor, pain comes in rhythmic, wave-like, "violent" (Lizette) contractions that pulse, agonize, shatter and overwhelm and then briefly disappear, providing women with respite, rest and moments of cohesion in-between the pain. The pains of labor are also productive and integral to the creative act of birthing new life. For many middle-class women who had homebirths, birth was constructed as a paradoxical experience involving both pain *and* enjoyment. Furthermore, in their narratives, pain had complex meanings and was not simply negative or something to be alleviated or eradicated as presumed in medical or phallocentric models of birth. Instead, there was often a deep satisfaction involved in wrestling with the paining body during labor. For example, Maggie made an interesting contrast between the intense pain of her satisfying homebirth experience and the pain-free but disappointing birth via epidural that she experienced in a local private hospital.

Rachelle: So this was the first time you actually did the whole thing without . . . ?
Maggie: Without a single painkiller (. . .) um, epidurals you just feel the pressure of the contractions and the pressure of the birth and it's uncomfortable, it's not sore, this was very, very sore (R: hmm) it was sore but the time, because you're focusing so much on breathing through the pain, the time goes much faster, lying in hospital, wai(ting) and watching your contractions, the time drags, you're just *lying* there, you're watching TV, you get bored because you're not actually active (. . .) his birth went so fast (. . .) it went, those, those 90 seconds of absolute agony disappeared like that, for a minute I was laughing and joking until the next—"***Oooh, the next one's coming***" (R laughs) and you lose it, for 90 seconds you actually, your head goes somewhere else, and then it comes back and then you're smiling at your friend again, and you're joking, until the next one hits you.

According to Maggie, the passive and pain-free laboring body produced by an epidural in (private sector) medicalized modes of labor was not a satisfying corporeal experience. She describes her self as sharply split off from her medicalized object-body—"you're watching TV, you get bored" while waiting and "watching your contractions." There is no embodied agency—"you're not actually active." In contrast, homebirth was "very, very sore" but involved a complex entangled duality of self and body (Akrich & Pasveer, 2004). Pain and pleasure were intertwined as part of the labor process, which veered between "laughing and joking" and "90 seconds of absolute agony." In this pendulum movement, Maggie is able to construct an active form of embodied agency that is experienced as deeply satisfying in her post-birth narrative. Chantelle, who gave birth in a public sector maternity unit, also described feeling more satisfied by her third birth in which she felt strong pains, but that proceeded without many medical interventions. For example:

Chantelle: With the others [births] I was always *laying* in X [public hospital], the, and there was lots of complications, my blood pressure was always, my blood pressure was always high (*) and um, they kept me there, two, three days (. . .) as I say I never got strong pains and they keep me in and then I must just lay and lay and lay (small laugh) (R: okay) but this one was like instant (giggles).

(Black, low-income, MOU birth)

Pain, satisfaction and pleasure thus sometimes involved complex entanglements in fleshy birth narratives. As opposed to other experiences of bodily pain (illness, injury, violence), pain during birth is normal, productive and associated with the creative generation of life. It is thus not surprising that the meanings of labor/birth pain are multiple and complex for women (see Klassen, 2001).

Telling distress

Fleshy pleasure tellings were stories of embodied agency, engagement, connectivity, and bodily resistance. There were, however, other kinds of fleshy tellings materializing in birth stories that did not reproduce pleasure, fun, satisfaction or enjoyment. I describe these as fleshy distress tellings and regard them as a form of 'chaos narrative' as outlined by Frank (1995). In chaos narratives, the storyteller is caught in the vortex of trying to tell a series of unending, overwhelming and distressing happenings for which there is no sense of overarching meaning or narrative order. Rather than coherence or satisfaction, in chaos narratives there is a gaping 'hole' that cannot be stitched or sutured. According to Frank (1995, p. 98), "the story traces the edges of a wound that can only be told around." I found that chaos narratives were rarely present in 'pure' forms in relation to birth but that they were often told in dialogue with other narrative types. For example, in women's accounts of elective caesareans, distress tellings often rode alongside medical restitution narratives and produced a narrative tension between (at least) two contradictory versions of events. Elective caesareans were thus told as both, "it was fine" (restitution) *and* as traumatic and distressing (chaos).

Women who experienced elective caesareans thus usually spoke in dual voices, telling a stable restitution narrative ("it was fine") while also telling a chaos story about the fleshy, lived experience of caesarean section ("it was horrible"). When spoken in this fleshy voice, caesareans were told as awful, weird and terrifying. In these narratives, the 'I voice' of the narrator was overwhelmed and overridden by a voice of chaos and medicalization. Women seemed to become "talked over and owned out" of their own stories so that, "even in speaking [they became] spoken for" (Pollock, 1999, p. 162). In fleshy distress tellings, the woman became, "the absent figure in her own story" (p. 162) as embodied agency disappeared and she became the disembodied object of bureaucratic procedures, surgical practices and medical interventions. The narrative of Hannalie best exemplified the dialogical tension/s involved in telling elective caesarean as both a classic restitution narrative ("I was fine, I had a caesarean and I was fine again") and as a chaotic, terrifying and distressing lived experience. The multivocality of her narrative is best represented in poetic form. The following narrative poem was constructed using techniques derived from the Listening Guide (see Gilligan et al., 2003) in which the movement of the 'I voice' is traced and foregrounded. The poem also traces the use of other pronouns in Hannalie's telling, such as 'they' and 'it,' and the 'and then' speech style identified by Frank (1995) as characteristic of chaos narratives.

High expectations

> I was very excited
> I was never nervous
> I was just excited
> I'd never thought
> I'm having an operation
> I just thought
> I'm having a baby

Bureaucracy (and having a birthday!)

> and then
> we booked in
> and
> and then
> they said
> then they come in
> and they
> and they
> in-between
> I was
> I was having a birthday!

Becoming a patient

> I was
> I was
> and then
> and then
> and they said
> and then
> and then, um
> and yes
> then

The surgical procedure

I started getting very excited
and then
they came
they put me on the trolley
and they took me
and then
they said
and then
and then
he injected it
then he did the spinal
and then
and then
I was in
and then
I started going numb
and um
then
and then
they covered me
and then
and
and then

Fleshy experience

I didn't know
I mean
I started going numb
you go numb immediately
I was under
I was going
I was
I went numb
I thought
you start feeling numb
you can't
I could
I could
but
but
I was

I couldn't
I couldn't feel
and then
I couldn't control
I was a dead pound of flesh

Voice of restitution

and . . .
<u>anyway</u>
but that was fine
it's not painful at all
it's just
it's weird

Fleshy experience

and then
I think
I might
I felt like
I started feeling sleepy
I thought
I'm not
I want
I'm completely aware
I can talk
but
I'm feeling
I had a bottle of wine
and (★) and
my breathing um (★)
I was breathing
I was like
it felt like
I was watching a movie
I was watching
I wasn't there

Voice of restitution

I won't do it any different
I'll still do it
I'd still rather do that

I now can know
I've been through it
but everything was fine

Fleshy experience

I said
I can't at all
I would
but I didn't <u>at all</u>
I didn't feel <u>anything</u>
<u>nothing</u>
I didn't feel at all
I must say
I dunno
I was a bit out of it
I think
I dunno
I could talk
but
I felt like
I'm breathing *slower and slower*
I'm thinking
"Am I going to die?"
"Am I gonna be okay?"
(laughs)

Voice of restitution

but everything was obviously fine

Fleshy experience

and then
they lifted him out
I was relieved
I didn't
I heard
I didn't know
and then <u>suddenly</u>
they lifted him up
and then
I only saw

I knew
I looked
<u>and</u>
<u>I dunno</u>
I looked
it didn't feel like
it was my baby

I looked
I thought
I don't know
I said
"Oh cute"
I said
I think
I think
I said
"Oh cute"

I was like looking
I smiled
and then
and then
and then
I could
I looked at him
I felt so weird
I felt like
I dunno

Voice of restitution

it was a very <u>fine</u> procedure
I mean
I was glad
I was
I was

Fleshy experience

but um
I dunno
it felt like
I was watching
I mean

and then
they took him
and then
I was relieved
I didn't want
I was not coping
I didn't feel
I was feeling horrible

Voice of restitution

I was
everything was fine
they said
I recovered

Fleshy experience

I started shaking
I started shaking
I didn't like that
my body went into shock
it was fine
I was just shaking
I wasn't cold
I was just shaking
I just wanted to become
a human being again
you know

I couldn't move
I had to
you can't move
it's too sore
you're lying there
it's bleeding
it's horrible
I thought
I dunno
I'm gonna
I'm immobile
I couldn't move
and then

Recovery and restitution

I
the next day
I got up
it was nothing
I realized
I got up
it was fine
I was fine
I walked
I put
I washed
I got
I got up and out
I was fine
I fed him
I changed him
it was fine
I got up
I felt better
I could
I looked
I spoke
it dawned on me
I requested
I said
I wanted
I was
I went

I
I
I said
I think
I took him home
<u>but I was fine</u>
I was fine.

Representation of long chunks of Hannalie's birth story in the form of a narrative poem shows her narrative as a complex entanglement between two contradictory storylines or narrative voices—namely, the voice of restitution: "it was fine" and the voice of fleshy distress: "it was terrifying and horrible." There is no singular story here but inherent multivocality and contradiction. According to Ochs & Capps (2001), narrative meaning-making often involves an inherent tension between our desires to 'fit into' a coherent, culturally acceptable storyline and to tell and trace the complexities of lived, bodily experience. Women telling elective caesareans were further torn between the desire to confirm their birth choice as 'right' and wanting to tell psychofleshy experience. As a result, in Hannalie's narrative an unbreachable 'gap' remained between contradictory storylines that was never sutured. Thus, despite her 'horrible' experience, she never rejected or eschewed medicalization but continued to reiterate that having an elective caesarean was the right choice. Her narrative thus does not make reflexive sense of why her lived experience was distressing or disappointing. As a result, "there is a hole in the telling" (Frank, 1995, p. 102), that traces around the unsutured wound of disappointment and loss.

Other women told 'purer' chaos narratives, in which distress and suffering were articulated more univocally. For example, Alison's private hospital birth, which was narrated as a cascade of endless interventions and disruptions, materialized as a classic chaos narrative in which she narrated the fleshy experience of labor/birth as one of being overwhelmed and over-run by medicalization. Similarly to several women giving birth in the public sector, Alison narrated the course of her fleshy birth experience as interrupted, and disrupted, by outside others. In the poem below, constructed from a section of interview transcript, Alison narrates her movement from embodied agency to chaos, loss of agency and being overwhelmed by medical others.

Embodied agency

it was *really* nice
I could still *feel*
it wasn't sore
I knew
I needed
I would know

Disruption and distress

but then
there was confusion
I was a bit in-limbo
and then
my contractions *slowed*
and they
they weren't as strong
and then
they started worrying
and then
he [doctor]

he put
and then
and then she [baby] was
and then
she was going

and then
he did
he put
it took effect
it went down
he did it
I was
she
it's *awful*

they
they've got
they put
they
they struggled
she was
she'd been
and then
you hear
and then
it went
I was trying
it was
it was horrible

and then
they said
he said
I should
you know
it was

I said
I
I couldn't understand *why*
I was
they
I mean
I couldn't understand why
I

they just
I had to
then
it happened
and then
I was struggling
I was crying
I just
I did
I
I was in tears
I didn't wanna go

and then
and then
it was *all go*
it was emergency caesar.

Alison tells of becoming overwhelmed by interventions, foetal distress, medical interruptions and loss of control, with her fleshy experience overtaken and consumed by medicalization. In the midst of medical chaos, she is unable to find support and affirmation from those around her. Instead, she *becomes* a victim as interventions spiral and she is bullied in/through a biomedical risk economy, which enacts repeated messages that her body is incapable and that she has failed at efforts to birth her own baby. In the public sector, women also narrated chaotic scenes in which their laboring bodies were constrained, interrupted and denigrated. In these narratives, the diminishment or 'muting' of fleshy experience was often enacted via both subtle and direct violations (see Chapter 5). For other women, the fleshy experience of labor and birth itself was inherently overwhelming and unmanageable. In these stories, women narratively performed a chaotic body, "swept along, without control" (Frank, 1995, p. 102), often unable to find support and recognition for pain and suffering. For example, Ophelia, who gave birth in a public sector hospital, told her story as if there was no way of escaping the onslaught of pain and fleshy chaos of labor/birth.

Ophelia: **Then** they [medical practitioners] felt *again* then they said I am *two* centimeters open but they said it can take a **long time**, the first centimeters you open *slowly* (R: hmm) but *that* was, I was, I was about two centimeters after two hours (R: okay), after another hour I was three centimeters, after another hour <u>and a half</u> I was *four* centimeters ^^then I STAYED four centimeters^^ and I did not open any further (*) after ten hours (**) yes, after I was in labor for ten hours, then they <u>broke</u> my water because they said ten hours is long enough, and then they <u>broke</u> my water (R: hmm hmm) I STAYED four centimeters, *my water* ran and *my water* ran and the pain exhausted me, they put me on *aaa,* um, the heart (inaudible) they put that on and monitored the child, they said the water is now broken, the child will COME (R: hmm), the child didn't come (*) and *the water* ran and **the pains** came and the waters ran—for *seven* hours <u>on and on</u>, now it's already 17 hours in labor (. . .) and then they explained to me what they were gonna do, they were going to *caesar* me and from my navel down, here at the bottom, I will be paralyzed and that, ***and then*** I was **scared** because it is *AN OPERATION* (R: hmm) and then they took me . . .

(Black, low-income, public hospital birth)

In this extract, Ophelia is caught up in an endless wave of happenings, which she has no ability to negotiate or control. While medical practitioners exert more active agency than she does ("they felt," "they said," "they broke," "they put me"), the fleshy 'body-in-labor' (Akrich & Pasveer, 2004), takes over and over-whelms the entire experience—"and *the water* ran and **the pains** came and the water ran." Constant references to "then" and "and then" function as a style of telling characterized by interruptions, in which each clause is cut off by the next. This speech style re-performs a lived, fleshy experience of chaos in which bodily events are without sense, order or coherence and one uncontrollable thing happens after another.

Fleshy chaos narratives were attempts to articulate the bodily and lived phenom-enology of distressing birth experiences. While these narratives were rarely 'pure,' and were usually told in dialogue with other narrative templates, the voice of chaos gives glimpses of the fleshy and experiential distress some women experience dur-ing labor/birth. As a result, these stories countered normative medical narratives that frame birth as a fleeting, insignificant and banal event that has no psychosocial relevance to women's lives. Women's efforts to voice distress during birth carry the seeds of potential subversion because the lived, fleshy experience of the birthing woman is put at the center of the birth narrative. Even while overwhelmed and rendered passive in the story of the distressing event, in telling the narrator carries the possibility of agency, reflection and renewal. While some women could make little meaningful sense of birth experiences that were overwhelmed by medicalized interventions or the dominating and violating actions of institutions and caregivers, others turned chaos into ethical and responsible action through the telling of birth narratives *as testimonies*.

Testimonial tellings

Stories are told by bodies that are themselves the living testimony.

(Frank, 1995, p. 140)

Experiences of distress were either told via fleshy chaos tellings or converted into testimonial narratives. Turning distress into testimony meant that birth events characterized by violation and mistreatment, were interpreted—not as a series of uncontrollable, contingent and meaningless happenings—but as *acts of wrongdoing*. Women telling testimonial narratives turned their birth stories into ethical actions in which they took a stand against mistreatment. Testimony is, of course, a very particular type of narrative telling and is usually associated with evidence given by an individual 'witness' in a courtroom or in religious settings (Park-Fuller, 2000). In classic testimony, the witness declares 'the truth' of what happened or what was seen (to a formal audience) and takes an active (and literal) stand in relation to a particular matter. According to Park-Fuller (2000, p. 22), testimony can be seen as, "a transgressive political act" that is used to counter dominant narratives (see also Pullen, 2015). Via the act of 'bearing witness' and taking an ethical position, the teller takes responsibility for 'making sense' of the event in question and countering injustice (Mohoto, 2015). In testimonial stories, suffering and violation have to be transformed, via reflexive action, from fleshy lived experience/s into narrative coherence. Testimonial tellings are thus inherently embodied and tied to the body (Frank, 1995; Pullen, 2015). They are also potentially powerful acts of narrative resistance, in which tellers take up a reflexive and subversive position in relation to power, acts of wrongdoing or violation. Testimonial narratives are also inherently dialogical acts, interweaving 'the truth' of past events with narrative modes of reconstruction and inevitable positioning/s against counter-claims and counter-testimonies.

Testimonial narratives were found to be a central mode of birth storytelling used by low-income women who had given birth in public sector settings. While I positioned the research study as a broad and benign exploration of 'birth stories,' several marginalized women 'read' or interpreted the study as being about mistreatment in public sector maternity services. As a result, without prior framing, women sometimes positioned themselves from the outset of interview encounters as 'taking a stand' against unacceptable treatment in public sector maternal health services. Women either took up positions that used their experience to confirm public sector mistreatment or countered this story. While the narrative invitation extended to women at the start of interviews asked them to 'tell what happened from beginning to end with the birth,' some women immediately set off by talking about acts of mistreatment or by noting that they had not experienced mistreatment. For example, Rosetta started her story in the following way:

Rosetta: I went in (*) before I gave birth I lay on the bed and then when I was finished giving birth then they um (*) they put the baby on me and (**) my afterbirth was still <u>inside</u> me (R: hmm) and then they went to help another mommy (R: okay) and then I lay for about two hours with the afterbirth inside me (R: okay). I told the counsellor that I was very upset about that, I was (**) **upset** (*)

(Black, low-income, MOU birth)

Rosetta starts her testimonial narrative by recounting a distressing and upsetting episode of mistreatment by health care workers in which she was left unattended with the placenta still inside of her. Her narrative then proceeds to tell of a series of mistreatments, all of which were framed in relation to injustice and wrongdoing on the part of health care workers. As she later said, "they don't treat you right," sketching events in which she was ignored, neglected and treated harshly and impatiently by nurses. The birth environment is described as one in which one couldn't even ask a question without fear of abuse. For example, "I wanted to ask her, the way she treated me did not even give me a chance to ask why I was bleeding." Rosetta's entire birth narrative is framed *in relation to* a wider community discourse of abuse and mistreatment in public maternity clinics. As she put it, "everyone complains about X [MOU], most of the mothers prefer to go to Y [public hospital]." This community discourse of mistreatment was thus found to frame and shape the birth stories of many low-income participants. Women, however, differed in how they positioned themselves and their birth experiences in relation to this storyline. For example, Rosetta took a stand to confirm the public narrative of mistreatment and offered her experience as evidence and validation of injustice and violations. She was also adamant that mistreatment was wrong and unacceptable. For example, when asked how the impatience and negativity of nurses might have made birth harder, she replied:

Rosetta: Yes, because why um (*) um she <u>chose</u> that work—to work with the babies and mothers, you have to have <u>patience</u> (**) you know? And she didn't have patience and that made me become, I was upset (R: hmm) cause I went home and I told the other mothers that I was going to report her, because the way she treated me was not right.

Towards the end of the interview, Rosetta's sister (Adelaide) joined in the conversation and chatted a little about her birth experience/s. According to Rosetta and her sister Adelaide, the nurses could not be 'bothered' to take care of women during labor. Consider the following exchange that illustrates the flow of local discourse about giving birth in public sector maternity clinics.

Adelaide: They would have, they didn't have patience, they wanted to um, the Flying Squad (emergency unit) came to take me, a young man and an old man (. . .) then the man told them off—"If we take her now for a caesar to X [hospital], then she will have the baby in the ambulance" #

Rosetta: Now that's what they do—they want to send the mothers for caesars because they don't have patience with the mothers (R: hmm hmm) they don't have patience, there by X [MOU] they must do something about the nurses at X [MOU] #

Adelaide: I was busy getting pains, I was lying on the bed, then they said they are going for lunch, they are now going to take lunch (R laughs) then they came back an hour later—what if I had had the baby? (R: Oh my goodness!)

Rosetta:	And they talk man
Adelaide:	While you are having pains
Rosetta:	They have conversations
Adelaide:	About what happened last night or they talk about the other nurses
Rachelle:	As if you're not there?
Rosetta:	Yes! It's like you're not even there (*) And if you call them perhaps and then they will tell you, you must just wait, we are not there, just wait, yes, they tell you that cause it's like (*) for them it's like YOU DON'T PAY for deliveries and stuff, you will just um accept whatever.
Adelaide:	But I read there—if any nurse doesn't treat you nicely, then you must talk to the manager—so . . .

According to Rosetta, "they must do something about the nurses" at the local MOU. She positions the nurses' actions as unacceptable and her own experience as part of a much broader pattern of mistreatment and injustice. Nurses are constructed via this dialogical exchange as impatient, careless and uncaring. The fact that women in the public sector do not pay for services is seen as one of the reasons why nurses treat them poorly. Furthermore, according to Rosetta, low-income women are also expected to, "just accept whatever" treatment they receive. This exchange also invokes rising community dissatisfaction with public sector maternity services and the circulation of a rights-based discourse in which women can/should report or speak up about incidents of abuse. Adelaide thus speaks about having "read there" (probably via posters at the MOU) that you can "talk to the manager" if you feel you have been mistreated. Entangled within public sector birth assemblages is thus a circulating community discourse about mistreatment and injustice, particularly within MOU settings. Women's testimonial tellings were thus told in relation to a wider narrative of injustice. Read optimistically, this could signal the beginning of a resistant collective movement among women against mistreatment and violation in public sector settings. The dissatisfaction, anger and righteous indignation expressed by some women in their testimonial tellings represent powerful affective energies that could be harnessed towards social protest activities.

Many low-income women that experienced distressing births thus reflexively enacted narrative resistance through the telling of their stories as testimonies of injustice. While they told of experiences in which they were muted, ignored and rendered passive, in/through a testimonial mode of telling they were able to construct themselves as active narrators, counter injustice and offer resistance. Vanessa, who gave birth at a MOU, initially responded to my narrative invitation to tell her birth story by framing events in relation to the clockwork narrative (see Chapter 3). However, she quickly adopted a testimonial telling in which she spoke out against practices at the local MOU.

Vanessa: I got pains and pains at home and then uuh the Thursday I got pains and then I went to X [MOU] and then they checked me out (*) then I was three centimeters and then they, I stayed there and uh (*) overnight there and then in the middle of the night they examine you again to see how far you are and that (R: hmm) and uh (**) uuum (*) in the morning then they check again to see how far you are (*) *but* the way I see it there, it's not right how they treat the people (R: okay) uuh . . .

(Black, low-income, MOU transferred to public hospital)

Vanessa starts out recounting the birth story in a standard fashion, using clocktime measurements. However, it is soon evident that this is not the story *she wants* to tell. She thus changes the direction of the telling and signals the start of her testimonial narrative by saying, "*but* the way I see it there, it's not right how they treat the people." Vanessa then proceeds to tell birth in relation to an over-arching testimonial narrative. For example, "there is no support, it's just you alone there," they don't care about the people, so (*) and the way the toilets look is disgusting," "a person gets nothing, nothing (. . .) not even a cup of tea or a piece of bread (. . .) nothing (*) nothing." She also repeated throughout her narrative that the way women were treated during labor/birth was "not right." Forced to adopt a passive position during labor in which she, for example, received no information and was sent to a public hospital in an ambulance with no explanation offered by health care workers—"they explain nothing, just they [ambulance] fetch you and then *off* you go," Vanessa was able to adopt an active and reflexive position and enact narrative agency via her testimonial narrative.

A testimonial style of narrative telling was strongly articulated by Tracy-Lee. Even before the interview began and the tape started running, she (and her family, who were also present) made it clear that the interview was important in allowing her a space to tell what she had experienced, and witnessed, at the local MOU. The family also told me that they had wanted to officially report the mistreatment she suffered, but because of fear of reprisal, they had decided not to. The interview thus offered them (and Tracy-Lee) a safe space in which to 'bear witness' to what had happened to her. What was also interesting about Tracy-Lee's testimonial narrative was that it included both an account of what happened to her, and what she witnessed happening to other women at the local MOU. Her experience was unusual because she spent three days at the MOU while she was ill with a kidney infection (which was misdiagnosed). As a result, she was able to 'bear witness' in a unique way to what she saw happening to other women that came and went while she spent time at the clinic. As a result, Tracy-Lee told a powerful and detailed testimonial narrative outlining the inhumane conditions and treatment that she witnessed (and experienced). As she put it, the way she was treated at the MOU made her feel "*like an animal*" and "like I wasn't there."

Tracy-Lee:	It was very upsetting for me, yes, especially the way they speak to the patients and scream at the patients in labor—keeping their legs open, forcing it open #
Rachelle:	So you had to, to witness—you had to see all of this happening?
Tracy-Lee:	Yes, and I saw, while this one girl was in labor she was also laying in her own vomit and they left her just like that (★) it was here by her arms and things and I had to see all of these things (. . .) the way they treat them [women-in-labor] and like ↑"Com(e), come, you wanted this, you wanted the child—*push, push!* Hold your legs"↑ and **forcing** the legs open, like one keep this one and one keep that way #
Rachelle:	So you had to watch—you had to see this?
Tracy-Lee:	I saw this (. . .) and it was *scary*, I was really, I was really afraid, I thought I'd rather give birth at home than suffer like that . . .
	(Black, low-income, transferred to public hospital)

She was adamant that the conditions and 'care' at the MOU were *unacceptable* and that strong action needed to be taken to sort out the problem.

Tracy-Lee:	I would really prefer that (★★) X [MOU] should be shut down actually, I don't think that (★★) place should exist cause I don't think those people are equipped to deal with such kind of things (R: okay, okay) they don't even have Panado [paracetemol] there. . .

Like Rosetta and Adelaide, Tracy-Lee also referred to a rights-based discourse to bolster her testimonial narrative. She also described noticing a poster outlining patients' rights displayed on the wall at the local MOU. As she put it:

Tracy-Lee:	At the MOU there's, there's a_lot that needs to be improved (★) especially the way they *treat* the patients, I mean they have this bill of rights and responsibilities up (. . .) but they're not following that code of conduct and then they have the audacity to put the number there that ↑you can↑ (R laughs) in case of any problems but they still treat the people like that.
Rachelle:	Okay, so they need to be accountable?
Tracy-Lee:	To what they're actually saying, because as soon as you come in there, it's like on the wall—big—on the wall, next to the breastfeeding poster and espe(cially) the treatment, the patients should be more *uuh*, the nurses should be more with the patients and the cleaners should do their work (R: okay).

Tracy-Lee's testimonial narrative took a clear ethical stand against mistreatment and functioned as a powerful act of resistance and 'speaking back' against oppressive and inhumane conditions in public sector maternity clinics. At all times, she spoke strongly and with passion *against* the violation of women during labor/birth. Through the telling of this testimonial narrative she was able to find a way to turn dehumanizing and traumatic treatment into a form of resistance.

As mentioned, the 'matter' of poor care and mistreatment was already circulating in communities as a public discourse or local narrative about birth in public sector facilities. Women told testimonial narratives *in relation to* this community narrative and adopted positions either confirming and validating this storyline or repudiating it. Some women, speaking in relation to this cultural storyline, were careful to report that they had not been poorly treated. Without prompting, these women also framed their experience in relation to the mistreatment discourse. For example:

> *Bonita:*   Then they broke my water because the pain was too bad, I couldn't stand it anymore, then they broke my water, after about *two* hours they broke the water, then she [baby] came (R: okay, okay) but it was a, it was a <u>nice</u> experience with my second one, with my second time I was also at X [MOU], they weren't rude, nothing, they treated me very well.
>
>   *(Black, low-income, MOU birth)*

Bonita adds a disclaimer to her story, namely "they weren't rude, nothing." Many of the women that explicitly repudiated the storyline of mistreatment, also constructed 'other' birthing women as 'problems' (and hence deserving of poor treatment). For example, Bonita went on to say:

> *Bonita:*   I think most of the time when they [nurses] are rude with the people, the people are first rude with them, them they also become rude (R: okay).
> *Rachelle:*   Can you give me an example of what it would mean to be rude to them?
> *Bonita:*   Like some people don't know how *to talk*, they start swearing and that, then the sister will also, it's not right, if you want respect then you must give respect (R: yes, okay) now some people don't understand that.

Similarly, Carmen was clear on the view that nurses were not the problem and that many women brought troubles on themselves by the way they acted during labor. As she put it: "it's *HOW YOU ARE* with the nurse" that determines the way in which you will be treated. This puts the onus on laboring women to act appropriately and respectfully and justifies mistreatment when women misbehave. Furthermore, Carmen was clear that certain *kinds* of patients were especially problematic.

> *Carmen:*   You get **rude** young girls, most young girls are ***rude*** (R: okay) especially when they were on drugs they just want <u>their way</u> (R: oh okay), you can't always have your way (R: okay) you must listen to the nurses, you can't be cleverer than them because they studied for that.
>
>   *(Black, low-income, MOU birth)*

The irony here was that Carmen was herself a young mother who was recovering from drug addiction. Tolerance and acceptance of poor care and abuse from health care workers has been found to be common in obstetric settings in the Global South (see Bohren et al., 2016). Beliefs about 'difficult' patients and 'problematic women,' defined in relation to broader sociocultural discourses, were thus found in the talk of women themselves. Many women therefore repudiated the community storyline of mistreatment and violation/s in local MOU settings, either by simply offering their own experience as counterpoint or arguing more strongly that women themselves were to blame for any 'trouble' that might occur. A wider community storyline of mistreatment and violation was therefore a vitalizing force in low-income women's birth narratives. Without prompting, women often positioned their particular birth experience in relation to this discourse. While some women reiterated normative medical storylines about 'difficult' patients as the source of trouble in maternity wards, others told their birth stories as bold and countering testimonies of violation. Via testimonial narratives, women were able to find a way of reflexively enacting narrative resistance by defining mistreatment as unacceptable and unjust.

Summary

This chapter explored narrative acts of countering, resistance and subversion. While some stories carried only the quiet and subterranean seeds of normative disruption (i.e. fleshy distress narratives) others burnt hot and loud in resistance against injustice (i.e. testimonial narratives). I argued that bodies are key to hearing subversion and alternative storylines. Resistance to normative storylines does not always materialize via fully formed or coherent narratives. Instead, possible points of disruption are often voiced as fleeting, inchoate or "strangled articulations" (Chadwick, 2014, p. 48) on the margins of hegemonic frames. Often resistance emerges 'between the lines' as fleshy eruptions in storytelling. As a result, bodies—often muted by normative narratives (i.e. biomedical) 'speak back' offering embodied resistance that materializes as the *excess* in language—laughing, sighing, babbling, stuttering, shouting, whispering and crying. While often seen as 'debris' (McKendy, 2006) in conventional approaches to qualitative and narrative analysis, my analytic approach was guided by being 'turned on' to the affective, fleshy currents of telling. As a result, I came to see how comedy and humor could function as modes of embodied resistance that poked fun at normative narratives and subverted their logic and assumptions. The laughing and giggling body spoke in the resistant language of humor to challenge the status quo and disrupt 'doom and gloom' stories of birth that focus on complications, horror and represent birth as a grueling ordeal. Enactments of comic subversive narratives also worked to position birthing women as the heroines of the birth drama and the center of the fleshy comedy of birth.

Modes of resistance also materialized in/through *the telling* of the fleshy labor/birth experience. While the psychofleshy experience of labor/birth is routinely muted in clockwork narratives and normative biomedical and phallocentic ontologies of birth, in women's tellings, the birthing body often *spoke back against erasure* via fleshy eruptions and embodied ways of telling. Without evoking 'the body' as external referent or 'object' in these tellings, women spoke the embodied pleasures of labor/birth through fleshy language vitalized by laughter, loud utterances, shouting, high-pitched articulations and sounds that worked to re-enact the exuberance of laboring/birthing corporeality. Importantly, while both middle-class homebirthers and low-income women articulated the fleshy pleasures of labor/birth, these tellings were more common among women giving birth at home. Enacting embodied agency and the fleshy pleasure/s of birth were not therefore free-floating forms of resistance, but were enabled by birth assemblages characterized by warm relations, connectivity and body-to-body support. As a result, it was usually only low-income women that gave birth in supportive, caring environments that were able to enact such forms of bodily agency, power and pleasure. While the fleshy pleasures of labor/birth were told via the excessive vitalizing force of speaking bodies, distress was also told as an embodied narrative marked by particular ways of telling. Fleshy distress was often told as a chaos narrative (see Frank, 1995), in which tellers were overwhelmed by bodily suffering and unable to find ways of making sense of their lived experience. While not overt forms of narrative resistance, fleshy distress tellings nonetheless were disruptive of normative narratives in that they tried to tell the lived corporeality of birthing distress. As a result, the embodied perspective of the teller was articulated, even if only in subterranean and hushed tones, and thus functioned as a counterpoint to normative storylines and discourses that collectively 'mute' the psychofleshy experience of birth.

While fleshy tellings of labor/birth often worked on the margins of normative narratives to disrupt, counter and subvert, there was another order of narrative resistance outlined in this chapter that was bold, loud and non-apologetically subversive. Interestingly, these 'loud' voices of subversion belonged to low-income women, who often took a strong stand *against* injustice and violation in their birth stories. These women, subjected to acts of violation and mistreatment during labor/birth were able to reflexively enact resistance in/through their birth narratives. Telling testimonies of violation enabled them to take up positions of agency and resistance after having suffered erasure, loss of agency and dignity during birth. These testimonial tellings and reflexive acts of resistance also materialized as part of a wider, growing community dissatisfaction with mistreatment and circulating rights-based discourses. Hopefully, these testimonies signal the beginning of a collective narrative speaking out against injustice that will spark and ignite a social movement of protest against the abuse of women during labor/birth in public sector services.

7

WHAT MATTERS?

Vitalizing birth politics

Birth is politically and morally contested and subject to competing idealizations, valorizations and ontological contestations. According to Reiger and Dempsey (2006, p. 364), there is a "sense of crisis around childbirth" in the twenty-first century. Debates about what kind of birth is best and what *matters* in relation to birth are fraught and volatile. Ideological warfare is being waged between obstetricians, midwives, activists, academics, mothers and birth workers about the meanings of birth, birthing bodies, femininity and birth justice. Rates of caesarean section and medical intervention are unjustifiably high across many global settings, many women are dissatisfied with maternity care, fearful of birth (Reiger & Dempsey, 2006; Nilsson, Bondas & Lundgren, 2010), traumatized and distressed by their birth experiences (D'Ambruoso, Abbey & Hussein, 2005; Swahnberg, Thapar-Björkert & Berterö, 2007; Cindoglu & Sayan-Cengiz, 2010; Schroll, Kjaergaard & Midtgaard, 2013; Nilsson, 2014) and rates of maternal and infant mortality continue to mirror global and local social inequalities in relation to race, class and geopolitics. The polarization between biomedical and 'natural' modes of birth and between physiological and technocratic birth continues to stymie birth politics and activism (Walsh, 2010). Birthing women are often the inadvertent losers in these birth wars and debates. Middle-class women are caught between idealizations of 'normal birth,' risk discourses, moral imperatives, fears over safety, the neoliberal promise of individual choice and concomitant burden of responsibility and the sociomaterial machinery of the 'medical-industrial complex' (Rossiter, 2017). Marginalized women are caught within multiple currents of sociomaterial forces and subject to stigmatization and structural disrespect in health care facilities on the basis of race, class and other identity markers. They also face the compounding effects of poverty, social marginalization and racism as they navigate maternity services during pregnancy, labor and birth.

The time is ripe to forge new lines of thinking that vitalize the feminist politics of birth. In order to improve maternity care for women and move beyond unproductive binaries, polarizations and idealizations, we need to begin by listening to what *matters* to women in relation to birth. The politics of birth can only be productively built on the bedrock of (diverse) women's perspectives. To this end, this book has attempted to weave together a heterogenous mix of voices speaking about birth from very different perspectives and sociomaterial locations. While earlier chapters focused on power relations and modes of resistance, in this chapter I explore how birthing bodies—the ways they were framed, enacted and treated—emerged as central to women's *feelings* about their birth experiences. I present a 'collective assemblage of voices' (MacLure, 2013) drawn from women's stories to begin to explore what matters to women in relation to labor/birth. What makes women feel 'good' or 'bad'? Can we trace continuities in what matters to women across multiple birth assemblages? In the context of heterogenous sociomaterial relations, race–class divides and structural differences, is the enunciation of a 'good birth' even possible? In this chapter, I am interested in exploring what happens when we put affective and fleshy bodies at the center of thinking about what matters in relation to birth/maternity care.

A collective assemblage of voices

In this section, I foreground women's voices and open up a fluid space focusing on their articulations of labor/birth. I do not present these voices as 'authentic' or regard them as representations of singularity or homogeneity. Instead, they are open, partial and emergent becomings, transversed and crisscrossed by multiple currents—including the fleshy body, sociomaterial ideologies, affective relations and the research matrix. What I am interested in here is the ways in which these voices might constitute a "collective assemblage of enunciation" (MacLure, 2013, p. 660) that both resists homogeneity—*and yet*—that also tells a flowing, weaving, multivocal story in which sticky sediments territorialize 'distressing' and 'good births' in particular directions. These voices thus stutter, leak and exceed neat categorization *and yet* they also speak in broad continuities about what matters to women in relation to labor/birth. I offer these voices as openings with which to begin to think about what makes women feel good or bad in relation to birth as a way of vitalizing birth politics.

Yolande (white, vaginal birth, private hospital)

> You lie there, totally exposed to the world
> Don't know what's going on
> I wasn't ready
> My body wasn't ready
> Every check up was painful

The gynae didn't understand
The labor was traumatic
Everyone's telling you what to do
And no-one's actually listening to you
It's all negative, there's no positive, it's all
It's guarded
You're just lying there
You get bored
The time drags
Your baby gets brought to you smelling of a Johnson's ad.

Janine (white, elective caesarean, private hospital)

I actually thought there would be a bit, a bit more
Dignity to having a caesar
But it's not
They will see everything from every angle
You are there for all to view (★) in all different positions
You're just like a doll there
They just do whatever they have to do
It's like you're basically not even there.

Cynthia (black, vaginal birth, public sector)

It was good
Because they talked with me
The one nurse talked with me
She said to me "push tigh-," the time when I couldn't push
I was TIRED
Then she said to me I must push
And then I **pushed**
They were <u>nice</u>, they *talked* with me
They were very nice
They weren't ru(de)
They didn't say *you* or IT
They were very nice
They *talked* almost like you are now (★)
You are <u>important</u>
It's *important* to them.

Sara (white, elective caesarean, private hospital)

I mean for the doctors
Like for them it's just another day at the office (laughs)
You know
It's not like a big deal

So they were chatting about
I think about golf or rugby at some point
And I was like
"**Please** this is an important moment—can we talk about this some other
    time?" (laughs)
Like talking about rugby and they're taking my child out
So—just pay <u>attention</u> all of you.

Tasneem (black, vaginal birth, public sector)

The **actual** birth
It was quite traumatic
You know
The **care** that was given wasn't what I expected
Especially with your first one
I, I gave birth prematurely, it was 33 weeks
They said
"Oh you're not supposed to be here, it's still eight weeks for you to go"
When they examined me
I was eight centimeters dilated
They had to call an ambulance
It was after an hour that they pitched up (sighing)
I was ten centimeters dilated
It was on the brink of the day shift turning into night shift
I suppose they were tired
They were saying 'Come on woman you must push the baby's head'
And you're first time
Not knowing what's happening
It was very much traumatic (deep breathing)
You don't know **what** to do
You don't know **how** to push

It was very much traumatic
I had to clean myself with this little **bucket**
They left me there all alone
Um, after they stitched me up
They told me 'Here's a bucket and you clean yourself'

I was actually very scared
There was no time for anything
I mean I just couldn't stop pushing (both laugh)
I had to <u>just push</u>
I couldn't cope
I forgot how to breathe
I couldn't handle it
So fast, it was so fast

I was very scared
I just couldn't stop pushing.

Angela (white, planned homebirth)

Through every contraction
They breathed with me
And held me
That made such a difference
For the pain
I dunno why
Every time one of them would go away
I'd feel the difference in pain.

Michelle (white, planned homebirth)

You're almost like all separate from your body in a way
Your head's here and
Your body's busy doing it's own thing
There was no spiritual element at all
It was very basic, very (⋆) um much more real this time round
There was no high of, my body sort of taking me, putting me on a different level
It was just,
It was quite real.

Phoebe (white, elective caesarean, private hospital)

I was just lying there
I couldn't see
You've missed things
You haven't
You haven't been aware
I mean it's, it's not a major issue
But
It's like things
You actually would like to know
It's frustrating
Um
But anyway . . .

Wendy (black, vaginal birth, public sector)

^^Nobody came^^
The pains got <u>stronger</u> and <u>stronger</u>

And um (★)
Then I went to one sister and *asked* her like (★★)
Won't she check on me to see how far I am
How many centimeters I am?
And um then she said
"*No*, um, do I <u>want</u> one, one of them to get **angry** with me?"
They are going to get **angry** and <u>scold</u> me
If I ask how many centimeters I am and that they must <u>check on me</u>
And then <u>um</u> (★)
Then I left it and then I went back to the room
Because I didn't want big trouble
Then I left it
And nobody checked me
And then (smacks lips)
Then I walked up and down
But they were cross about *that* as well
And said "*no* ^^I mustn't walk up and down^^" (laughs)
It wasn't a nice experience for me *there*
It wasn't at all nice.

Hannalie (white, elective caesarean, private hospital)

It was
The whole thing about it that wasn't nice for me
Was the fact that
I couldn't control my body
I was a <u>dead</u> pound of (★) <u>flesh</u> you know
There's no feeling whatsoever
To be quite honest
It felt like I was watching a movie
I was watching this all happening around me
But it wasn't
I wasn't there
I didn't feel <u>anything</u>
<u>Nothing</u>
I didn't feel at all
I'm thinking
"Am I gonna die?" "Am I gonna be okay?" (laughs)
but everything was obviously fine.

Joni (black, vaginal birth, public sector)

There was a monitor
There was the doctor

Here I was lying
I was facing the monitor and the doctor
And he was basically saying
"Oh okay, you're getting a contraction now, so start pushing"
I didn't feel a single thing.

Sheryl (white, elective caesarean, private hospital)

It was horrible for all my, my expectations
The anaesthetist
He walked in and *flung* his notes on the, on the bed
And the theatre's freezing
So I have this warm reception from the anaesthetist—
He was either having a really bad day or something
I think actually he shouldn't have been such a sh★t
Anyway
And it was the cold
And it was the insecurity
And it was his rudeness
And there was a lot of rushing around in theatre
And I just sat there and the tears just started to roll

It was really very impersonal
Because you're very sensitive
I was particularly sensitive
I think first-time moms are
The room was very cold
It was very cold for me

I could feel the pressure
But I couldn't feel the pain
So I said to him [anaesthetist]
You know um I can still move my feet—do you know?
And he says {Shall I tell you a secret?}
He says {We're not operating on your feet}
Which is funny now but at the time I (★)
And he says "You know what? We're halfway through"
So how would I know?
He thought he was very clever
With his little comments.

Sarayda (black, vaginal birth, public sector)

I had privacy (★) um
The nurses were very attentive um (★)
They were there all the time <u>for me</u>

Not leaving me alone
It was a good birth for me.
They were good with me
They gave me **excellent** treatment
<u>I felt good</u>

When I gave birth to her
And then I just asked the nurses to pray with me for her
And the nurses were standing there
They were so like um
They were really part of everything there with me

The *pregnancy* thing and the *birth* thing
I wanted to experience it as <u>natural</u> that I could
So when I sat down and
I felt this <u>guuussh</u>
Like this
I actually felt the bubble in my stomach—it opened—it burst
And that was <u>so nice</u>
And the water *came out*
I'm like "Wow! This is so nice!"
The experience for me was <u>beautiful</u>
I really *experienced* pregnancy because of the
My water that <u>broke</u> and my contractions coming like that
I knew exactly how to do it
<u>For myself</u>
Without anybody telling me

I felt like a <u>celebrity</u> there
The treatment they gave
It was very
It was very nice the treatment they gave me
Checked every time is my pillows okay
How are you feeling?
Checking my pulse and damping my head from the sweat and all of that.

Constance (black, vaginal birth, public sector)

They said I must go to the back
And then I sat there and waited
Then the pains came
Five hours
Then came the pains
Till ten 'o clock and then
I shouted
I called them

And they didn't worry
They just talked
Had conversations
Then when it was ten 'o clock I screamed
And then
I said it's burning
And then they came
To check how many centimeters I was
Then they saw
Then they said I must stand up to give birth
I was screaming the whole time
Then they shouted at me
I screamed because it was <u>burning</u>
And then she said
The one sister
"No, shut your mouth—why are you screaming? You scream because . . ."
Wait now?
^^Yes, "You scream^^ because you want to do such things" [have sex]

Rosetta (black, vaginal birth, public sector)

After I gave birth
My afterbirth was still <u>inside</u> me
And then I lay there for one or two hours
With the afterbirth inside me
I was very upset about that
I was um (**) **upset**
I was uncomfortable cause um (*)
The, the, the, the midwife she was very um (*)
<u>Impatient</u>
They don't give you a <u>chance</u> to, to to push the baby out
They, they, they want everything to just go <u>quick</u>
That's how they are
She was very frustrated (**) impatient and frustrated
I basically gave birth alone
I shouted
Then they look like that (*)
And then she just said I must push, push
Then she walked off again
I basically gave birth alone which um
There should have been someone with me
To help me and—you know?
But there was nobody.
The way she treated me
I didn't even have a chance to ask about the bleeding

Because I wanted to ask
I was scared
I was scared I was going to lose the baby because of the blood
I was upset about the treatment
They talk
While **you** are having pains
They have conversations
It's like you're not there.

Esther (black, emergency caesarean, public sector)

They were very nice
I wanted to buy a bunch of flowers for the one (both laugh)
They were very nice, <u>very nice</u>
I was on my *N-E-R-V-E-S* ^^but they were just nice^^ (laughs)
She was nice with me
She said to me
"Don't worry, it goes quickly, it goes quick"
Then she said
She was going to inject me
She, **she warned me** about the needle that she was going to use
{So yes, she was very nice} {very nice}
Everything was, I
I miss ^^those days at the hospital^^ (both laugh)
It was like a holiday for me, it was nice
There was nothing that was bad.

Beth (white, elective caesarean, private hospital)

I was being sewn up
And then
I must say
That was horrible
You're just lying there
Your baby's taken away
You're lying there as if
Okay well—*I'm* the one who produced this baby
and now (★)
everybody's ^^running about^^ (both laugh)
It's like you're there and going
"Fine, all right, is this it then?" (laughs)
So it was horrible
I felt
I felt
Very let down.

Tracy-Lee (black, emergency caesarean, public sector)

I was left alone
There was no one to mon   itor me
I vomited in the toilet
I was told to clean my own vomit up with tissue paper
And I *was so* sick
I couldn't even walk
Nobody came to come monitor me (intake of breath)

There's a lack of um pillows
There's no pillows at all
You had to sleep on your arm or bring your own pillows
They don't give you food there (★)
No food
Only in the morning coffee
Of which they've got two cups that <u>all the patients</u> must *share*
And there's about six beds in the *uuh*, <u>maternity</u> room
And then there's eight beds in the postnatal ward
And there's only two cups that people must share in the morning
And they give you two <u>dry</u> biscuits with that
You must bring your own food otherwise you're gonna *suffer*
And then there's lack of blankets as well
There was only about three of us that had blankets

One lady couldn't take the pain
They didn't help her
Nothing
They just told her to walk it off
And her water broke <u>in</u> the toilet
And it was lying there till the next morning
And there was a cleaner on duty
But it wasn't cleaned up
It was left there in the toilet
And blood stains and things like that
It was really <u>disgusting</u>

I felt . . .(★)
I <u>felt</u> like
Like an animal
That's (★) to talk the truth
Like I was (★)
I mean
If that was their passion then they would take better care of the patients
<u>But they didn't do that</u>
They left me like that

I could've stayed at home and
I would've got much better treatment
Cause it was like
<u>I wasn't there</u>
I see that they don't have respect for the other people also (★)
Especially if you're not married and things like that and you're just a teenager

And, and **there's no privacy**
Like the curtains is open
And your partner is allowed in only when you give labor (★)
When you're actually giving birth
And
It's like <u>no privacy</u>
I can look at the next woman <u>right next to me</u>
And I'm here with my partner
So there's no privacy
It's really disgusting
It was *scary*
I was really
I was really afraid
I thought I'd rather give birth at home than suffer like that (★★)
I just wanted to come home.

Erin (white, planned homebirth)

The, the pleasantness of the environment made a big difference
Just like being able to dance around in my bedroom
And then *afterwards* (★) getting back into <u>my</u> bath and having a bath
And then being tucked up <u>in my bed</u>
I mean you're in your own comfortable bed
And not a hard, hospital bed
It's just, it just felt <u>nice</u> (★) it was very lekker [nice]
Every time a contraction came I sort of grabbed him [partner]
I would kind of lean on him
And he said
He could feel how
How intense the contractions was by how heavy I felt (both laugh)
It's a very intense *physical* experience (★) and <u>it's work</u>, you know
<u>I feel very proud of myself</u> (giggles)

Bronwyn (black, vaginal birth, public sector)

It's very nice there, I felt like I was in ^^<u>a hotel</u>^^—*being served* (laughs)
It's nice there
They treat you <u>very well</u>
In the morning they come in and <u>greet you</u>

With a smile on their face and it's nice
And they always <u>talk to you</u>
Like make conversation
And so you're never lonely there
Or feel like you're **out**, you don't fit <u>in</u>
They're so nice and friendly
They were very supportive
They told me what *to do* and they weren't like
^^in a rush^^
They told me to relax also and (*) they were very <u>*nice*</u> (laughs)
It was, it was a nice *experience*
When she was born
Oooh ^^it was the best time of my life^^ (laughs)
It was all a, all <u>an experience</u>, all the *feelings* in one –
Happy, sad, emotional
Uuhh! It was <u>nice</u>.

Shiyaam (black, vaginal birth, public sector)

My <u>boyfriend</u> couldn't come in with me
So I was <u>alone</u> and I was a little bit (*) SCARED
Mostly I was **scared**
Because I was alone and the nurses <u>there</u> *are* (*)
They are not so nice
^^They are not so nice^^
it was **scary**
because there was <u>no one</u> with me and I didn't know *what* was going to happen
Will something be wrong with my child or (**)
Will something go wrong during the 'process'?

They said he [boyfriend] couldn't come in
He could only come when the baby was going to 'deliver'
Then they would call him
^^**but** it was **cold**^^ <u>that</u> night and then he *went*
<u>Serenity Fields</u> is a very rough place
Gangsters and that
They <u>shoot</u>
Then they [boyfriend and brother] *went home*
So he wasn't there
And then ^^I was <u>alone</u> and in a state and SCARED and *shouting*^^
The fact that **nobody** was *there* with me—that was—for me (**) **hard**
And it was for me
it made me more SCARED than *anything else*
Because nobody was with me
And I could see there is

when I came in there was a mommy with one of the (★)
The mommy was with her daughter
Then I thought that could be <u>my</u> mother there ^^with me^^
seeing they wouldn't let my *boyfriend* in
the mother held her hand tight and her mother *comforted* her
and that
but I didn't have ***that*** ^^opportunity^^ to be comforted
they just said now you must <u>push</u>
how did your mother pushed you out must you also <u>push</u>
I was angry with them—scared also.

At home when I started getting pains –
My *boyfriend* was sitting with me (★)
He helped to (★★) not take the pain ***away*** but he helped me
Rubbed my back and that
So he made it easier for me actually
When I was ***there*** [MOU]
I was alone and the pains were getting worse
and then I cried (short laugh)
And it was **sore**
and there was **no one**.
They [nurses] are rude and <u>scold</u> and I am not used to
It's was my first baby and I didn't expect
It to be ***such*** an experience
I was very scared—excited to see my baby
But SCARED because nobody was with me
and I was ALONE
and they were rude
Scolding—^^ "she nags," "nags" they say—and "lie flat" ^^
And then they said again
I must **lie still**
So they, they mostly just scolded.

Jane (white, planned homebirth)

It was **lovely**
I felt very supported
And it was good (★★)
And then things **really, really, really** got sore (laughs)
I was able
It's just pain and (chuckles) it's going to pass
And it **will** get better
I got my bottles of juice with flower essences and
I drank that
And that was **good**

And my husband was **there**
By then I was grunting and groaning
I wasn't quiet anymore
But it was quite good also
It helped to be able to give a good groan if I needed to
And um
And then
I had a **really, really** big contraction
And my waters broke
You could **see** it actually break
It was so forceful
I just
It knocked me **back**
It was so **intense**
This (★) push and the intensity
The pain intensity went *through the roof* . . .
I could just feel the, the, the first beginnings of this
Incredible pushing force
It just absolutely knocked me
I was on my back
The force of it
It was these **huge** waves of pushing, just . . .
It wasn't **me** pushing
It was such a force

So it was, it was a **fantastic** birth
It was really thrilling
It's the best thing I've ever done in my life!!
There was a lot of pain
But it was **so**, it wasn't traumatising **at all**
Ja, it was *really* **good**
In fact I really ^^want, want to have another one now to see if I can do it
   all again^^
Yes, it was, it was a **good** birth.

Madiha (black, vaginal birth, public sector)

They didn't take note of us
They did their own thing
<u>Walked away</u>
Went and sat there <u>on a couch</u>
Far away from us
Went and sat <u>on a couch</u>
And **then**

Then I felt the baby's head is going to come
Then I wanted to walk to them
But I couldn't
{I couldn't walk}
Then I screamed
"Sister, the baby is coming!"
Then she said
"No, go and lie on the bed man, the baby isn't coming now!"
And then (★)
Then I said to the other woman
"Go and tell the sister the baby is coming out now"
Because the head had already come out
Then she went and told them
And then they came running (★)
Then they got their stuff together

I asked, I asked
I asked them
Can't they make that thing *looser*
Because the pains come at the back and that thing
Is *tight, tight, tight*
And then
They said
No, that thing is there to monitor the baby's heart and all that
It was *very*, very uncomfortable
I couldn't even walk because
{*The drips were here in my hands*}
I would have liked to have walked
Because when you got pains you couldn't sit up
You couldn't lie on your back
Because then that thing then he makes
Then he **scratches** and stuff
That thing that does that man
He scratches the whole time on the page
Now you can't lie on your back
You must lie on your side the whole time so that
That thing can (★) monitor (★) the baby

And then
When the baby was going to come out
Then there came *two*
I don't know if they were students
Because the one, the one did the thingie [examination]
And then she said

Then she said
"Come, come, come, come"
Then she said in English
"Come, you must *open* your legs
You mustn't hold yourself stiff"
So she said to me
And then she said
Um as the pains come—in *English* she said
"As the pains come, then you must push"
And they just *stood there* and held your legs open
And then, then, then (★)
Then I <u>pushed</u> (★)
Because they were very rude.

Sam (white, vaginal birth, active birth unit)

I was actually full of jokes and stuff the whole labor
I was making jokes
And singing along with music
Even through contractions I was
My sister organized some nice mixed tapes
And I would sing along to the music
And then even on the pushing out stage
We played music
I was just trying to sing with it, because then you're relaxed
I remember the people laughing at me because I was singing too loud (laughs)
I was very strong you know.

Alison (white, emergency caesarean, private hospital)

They left me *completely*
Eventually I said to her [midwife]
You know, I don't know *what's* happening,
Can't you do a check <u>now</u>?
I couldn't understand why, everything was
I was nine and a half centimeters by this stage
Everything was all go
They could feel her head
I couldn't understand why I
They wouldn't let my body do the rest
Why I had to have this extra stuff?
Everything was happening and
I felt like my body was working and it knew what *to do*
It was
It's *really* disappointing.

Yolande (white, planned homebirth)

It's, it just makes you feel
A whole lot of different things
It's like a "I did it" kind of proud thing
It's a warm feeling cause
I
I
It was one of the best experiences
I've ever had

Somebody was holding my hand
Somebody was talking to me
Somebody was rubbing my back
Somebody was massaging my lower back
It was just the fact that there were people around who, who <u>cared</u>
And that <u>touch</u>, you know
I was in the middle of a contraction
Paula [assistant midwife] just put her hand across my back and just pushed gently
And you focus on the warmth of the massage
as opposed to the white pain of the contraction
It just makes
It makes it so much easier

It's not very dignified (★) I just kept thinking
I'm going to have to clean this floor
I kept laughing and saying
"This is not dignified girls, this is not dignified"
I'm messing all over
But with all the sheets and everything
you're not actually messing the floor itself
In hospital you don't see any of that
You're in stirrups
You're in green towels
What you see is the end product—the baby
Whereas when you're at home and you're squatting and (★) it's
It's not very dignified
It's messy
And there's water
And there's (★)
And there's blood everywhere
And it's not dignified
But um
It definitely helped to be
To be able to move around
Your body tells you exactly where it needs to be.

Janice (white, planned homebirth)

It was quite nice to have somebody there who was having a conversation with
    me between contractions (laughs)
And actually
It was quite bizarre
Because we'd be having a conversation and I'd have a contraction
And then resume the conversation (both laugh)
So I was like not focusing
It helped a great deal cause
I wasn't focusing on the contractions
And the pain
And all that
I was listening and participating in a conversation (laughs)

Roxanne (black, vaginal birth, public sector)

She was **rude** <u>with me</u> (*)
Because I hadn't brushed my teeth
And then she said
I mustn't talk in her *face*
Because my mouth <u>stinks</u>
And I must not throw my clothes on the ground
But I put my clothes <u>nicely</u> on the ground
Because there was no chair to put them on
Then she asked—
Am I so <u>messy</u> at home as well?

Lizette (white, planned homebirth)

They helped me out of the bath and
I became aware that these two midwives were drying me
With these towels
And they were both like kind of drying my legs
So it was as though they were kind of *kneeling* almost
In a way
And I was so
It was such an amazing experience
I mean
I really felt that <u>these women</u>
Who were taking *care* of women with humility and <u>with respect</u>
Aagh
It was just
I mean it was *so* powerful
I
Nobody's ever *dried* me—being an adult

Never mind going down on their *knees* and <u>two</u> women
Like kind of *drying* me
You know
And your body's
You're *bleeding*
And you're dripping stuff
And you're not like in the greatest shape
And they
They're like <u>there</u> with all your shit and everything
That was *so* special
That was really, really so special.

She [midwife] knows exactly what the contraction feels like
She knows exactly where you are
On the peak of it
She knows exactly what to tell you to help you deal with it better
How to breath you know
Like encouraging you in such subtle ways
Like if it's a really strong contraction she goes
"*Oh this is a great one*" you know
Like
"Go *fetch* it"
And so you like get into that
There's no way I could have done it without her
No way
On a practical level and kind of a support level
And like
You *need* to be with somebody you <u>trust</u>
You need to be in an environment that you trust
You can't be worried about
"How long is it taking?" or
The noise that somebody's making *outside* or you know
What conversation they're busy having
I mean
I can't remember a conversation anybody was having
I don't think anybody dared to talk

You see it was also going with support hey
I mean if you imagine the scene with Pete [partner] behind me
And I'm standing
And my sister's on
At my left leg and
The midwife's at my right leg and
My foot was actually <u>on</u> them
On their laps or something
My feet wasn't on the ground cause

I kept slipping on the ground
For some reason
So they held my feet
And then there's another midwife who's there next to the other midwife
Like say in the middle
And I'm standing
And then I would
Then I would feel the contraction come and then
I would go down
And I would say "Okay, it's coming"
And then
You would have everyone's energy and everyone's attention
Like on you
Yes, and it would be "*aaauuh*" amd everybody's "*aaauuhing*" with me
And you know
So they're *all* like right <u>there</u>
It's not like just
Kind of me sitting pushing like somewhere
Everybody's making *a noise* as well
So I didn't feel like <u>I</u> was grunting or anything
Like everyone was kind of grunting with me.

Tasneem (black, planned homebirth)

It didn't feel as if I just went through birth
I mean
You could still feel the pain but everyone was just smiling and chatting
And it was just, you know, doing your own thing
At your own time
It was just absolutely wonderful
Absolutely wonderful
When the people came—in the evening we had family come—
"Why are you smiling?" "Did you just give birth now?"
I said
Yes I did
But everything was
I just felt so energetic because there was no <u>pressure</u>
Um
Everything was just so serene and you know, romantic and tranquil
And it just, it just made <u>me</u> <u>feel good</u>
It made me feel <u>good.</u>

Fadwah (black, vaginal birth, public sector)

<u>She helped me</u> but she wasn't so supportive (★)
Like a nurse should be

She was just so—neverminded—just (★) <u>**so**</u>
Like I had struggles with my, with pushing
And she could've at least just (★) encouraged me
And say something like
'It's almost'
when it's out you know 'It's over'
And no, she wasn't
She was rather um (★★)
She said um
"This child is playing with me" [cross voice]
"I don't have time for children who play" [cross voice]
Something like that
And while I was struggling
She was walking around and doing <u>her stuff</u>

And um, like I was pushing
I was moving on the bed
Because of the plastic that was on the bed
And **I didn't notice** I was moving
Like she told me I must lay straight (★)
And I didn't know that I was like moving (★)
And then **she shouts** and then she say
"Lay straight, why are you laying that way?" (cross voice)
and I just left her
I just didn't take note
about them shouting or being rude
^^because of the pains^^
I just did my own thing

And before that there was another lady (★)
I messed on the floor (★) with the blood
Because I was pushing (short laugh)
She was there in the office
Now I was messing and she told me um, um
"Go and fetch a mop and clean up your mess"
She told me so and
I was just looking at her.

Lola (white, elective caesarean, private hospital)

It was a very positive experience
That moment that they lift her up
It's like everyone's sort of keeping their breath in
It's a fantastic moment
I think I could experience it better
Because I wasn't in pain
I was totally satisfied and fulfilled with, with what I went through

It was a fantastic moment
And um, all the doctors and the nurses and everything
They actually
They give you that moment
It's not as is if there's rushing around
It's uh made more special because they see you as a little family
It's not as if they're just there to do their job
So it is
That makes it very special
I think.
The anaesthetist was actually talking to me
Telling me what they were doing
What was going on and saying
"Ooh they're pulling him out, the head's coming out" and "ooh there's the
    baby!"
The tears were like rolling down my face (both laugh)
It was an *incredible* (★) um moment
It's really <u>amazing</u>.

René (black, emergency caesarean, public sector)

It was
It was very nice (★)
They attended you straight away
Helped you onto the bed um (★)
The um (★) what do you call it—that belt—the monitor
^^*Put it round*^^
And then I lay on the bed for a few *hours*
And they examined
They always gave me the centimeters
They were nice
They explained **what they were doing** and so on
And why they were doing this or that
^^It was nice^^ (laughs)

Towards an embodied and affective politics of birth

What emerges from this collective weave of voices? What do these voices tell us about what makes women feel good/bad in relation to birth? What kinds of birthing bodies become or are vitalized in women's tellings? How do ontological frames come to matter? In this section, I attempt to weave women's voices into a vitalized politics of birth based on my interpretations of *what matters* to women. I argue that dualist and polarized framings of birth (i.e. 'normal' versus biomedical; biological versus social), idealizations of particular modes of birth as 'authentic,' empowering or morally superior, and denigrations of technology and interventions as inherently disempowering, do not speak to what matters to women.

In/through this collective assemblage of voices, birth is enacted as a heterogeneous and emergent becoming that cannot be reduced to singularity. Birth is not a 'pure' event that can be separated into different 'parts'—i.e. this part physiology, that part culture. Birth is also not an event that can be divided up into a discrete set of 'factors'—i.e. 'control,' 'expectations' and 'support.' Fundamentally, birth is not the experience of a disembodied or even 'individual' self. These voices enact birth as a 'mangle,' swirling with affective currents, fleshy excesses, intercorporeal and cyborg relations and transaffectivity. Birth is not a static physiological or biological process that unfolds from the inside and that engages an individual body as its field of play. Instead, birth is enacted in these tellings as a spreading, seeping and expansive set of relations involving many bodies, configurations of power, objects, frames, ideologies, energies and sociomaterialities. Within this swirl of energies, bodies and practices, women are either able to enact forms of connection and affirmation or are reduced to isolation, loneliness and disconnection. As a result, women's voices teem with intense and varied feelings about their births—i.e. fear, excitement, confusion, anxiety, trauma, joy, enlargement, loss, loneliness, happiness, dehumanization and community. These feelings provide important insights into the sociomaterial arrangements and ontological politics of birth and must be the starting place for the vitalization of birth politics.

What matters? The affective politics of birth

The collective voices show that affective assemblages matter in relation to birth. What emerges as important to women is not necessarily type of birth (i.e. vaginal, caesarean, non-medicated or technocratic) but the kinds of affective energies, flows and relations circulating with/in particular birth assemblages. Stories of enlargement, pleasure and happiness do not reside in either the absence or presence of technology or interventions or in a 'type' of birth but involve the ability to enact embodied presence, agency and involvement and be connected to others in affirming, empathic and body-to-body ways. A 'good birth' is thus not necessarily a birth without medical intervention, technology or a so-called normal delivery. Instead, it is the affective energies and dynamics emergent in the sociomaterial birth experience that either enact marginalization or enable positive affirmations of self (see Lyerly, 2006).

In women's tellings, it was the sociomaterial arrangements between bodies, meanings and machines, vitalized by ontological politics, which enabled or disabled affirming connections with others. Technocratic interventions had no inherent meaning (i.e. a caesarean section or EFM)—instead, objects, machines and surgical practices *became meaningful* in relation to sociomaterial environs, ontological framings and their realization in/through affective enactments. Thus, a caesarean section could be experienced as alienating, disconnecting and objectifying (i.e. see Hannalie, Phoebe, Sheryl, Sara and Janine), a moment of relational presence and engagement (i.e. see Lola) or as a safe and reassuring procedure (i.e. see Esther). Many women in this study did experience caesareans as alienating experiences. This is not because caesareans are inherently disempowering or disconnecting but because of the onto-relational assemblages within which caesareans are often enacted. These are usually highly medicalized spaces in which the embodied personhood of pregnant women is disregarded and the ethical, political and social significance of birth is not recognized, valued or respected. In instances where practitioners actively include women in the caesarean procedure and treat the process of birth respectfully, caesareans can be experienced as affirmations and 'good experiences' (see Lola). Thus, caesareans *can* potentially be enacted in ways that affirm women, if the relational, ontological and affective matrix of 'medicalization' is reorganized. Similarly, an EFM is not inherently 'bad' or constricting. The articulation of this technology as disempowering or enriching depends on its framing, application and implementation by hands vitalized with/in affective economies and positioned within a wider ensemble of practices and relations. Thus, for Madiha, the EFM became constraining and disabling because it was enacted within an objectifying assemblage that disregarded her and treated the machine as more important than the birthgiver. On the other hand, René experienced the EFM as reassuring because it was administered within a warm and affirming ensemble of relations.

It is interesting to note the frequency with which women articulate their births as 'good,' 'nice,' 'lovely' or as characterized by feelings of 'warmth.' 'Good' feelings about birth emerged as products of affirming and supportive birth assemblages. In her brilliant essay, Lyerly (2006) argues that it is not mode of birth, interventions or place of birth that make a birth good, violent or distressing. Instead, it is, "the affective attunements" (p. 102) emergent in the birth experience that can reinforce marginalization, disempowerment, violation and negative feelings (shame, diminishment) or enable positive affective affirmations (joy, self-worth, confidence). To vitalize the politics of birth we need to recognize the importance of the relational, embodied and affective contexts in which women give birth. Women who felt 'good' about their experiences articulated birth as a fundamentally relational event as they described conversations, body-to-body support, the presence of others and small acts of embodied concern and encouragement. Supportive others were active participants *with women* during labor/birth—they were available and present both bodily and emotionally. Lyerly (2006) argues that a 'good birth' "begins not with location or technology, doctors or midwives, but with the emotional lives of women" (p. 109). This shifts emphasis away from the characteristics and outcome of a particular birth to the relational and affective context of labor/birth. It also moves attention away from the individual psychological characteristics of particular women to the affective assemblages in which they give birth.

Women who felt 'bad' or distressed about their births used words such as 'not nice,' 'traumatic,' 'horrible,' upsetting, scary and disappointing to describe their experiences. Central to these negative feelings was an overwhelming sense of lack of care. These voices collectively and repeatedly spoke about *becoming invisible* during labor/birth—"it's like you're basically not even there" (Janine), "it's like you're not there" (Rosetta), "I wasn't there" (Tracy-Lee). In some birth assemblages, affective relations were characterized by lack of concern and embodied care. In public sector contexts, this meant that women were left alone unmonitored and without medical care while in some private hospital settings, medical experts got on with the business of surgery and interventions but did not bother to make women feel part of proceedings. For different reasons, women were left feeling unimportant and invisible. Many women that felt 'bad' about birth spoke of negative and violent verbal interactions with others as dominant features of their experiences. As noted by Thomson and Downe (2008, p. 268), distressing births were thus not necessarily related to mode of birth but "to fractured inter-personal relationships with care-givers." Anger, impatience, disrespect and rudeness were imparted via hostile utterances, ugly words, mocking, shouting and the corporeal ways in which things were said and done (i.e. rough handling, grabbing, forcing, throwing things). Disrespect for the process of birth and birthgivers also materialized in/through structural conditions in public sector services (i.e. dirty conditions, no pillows or blankets, lack of food and no privacy) and made women feel bad. According to Ahmed (2014), emotions are not inside or outside selves but rather circulating currents that effectively create surfaces, boundaries and objects. She argues that, "the surfaces of bodies 'surface' as an effect of the impressions left by others" (p. 10). Emotions are moving affective currents within assemblages but they also involve sediments of attachments and investments—they "accumulate over time" (p. 11). As a result, bodies and objects become 'sticky' and "saturated with affect" (p. 11). According to new materialisms, it is these moving affective currents that *are* power relations. Thus, "power is not seen as something outside or beyond the flow of affects in assemblages, but *as* this flow itself" (Fox & Alldred, 2017, p. 27; emphasis in original).

Highlighting the centrality of the affective landscape/s of labor/birth (rather than simply type of birth or physical outcome) is an important step towards vitalizing birth politics and thinking about improving maternity care. According to Darra (2009), we need to recognize that what is most important in relation to birth is not the attainment of 'normal' birth but caring, respectful relations and the establishment of a trusting, affirming, dignified and respectful birth environment. This is an important shift given the unpredictability of the physiological processes involved in birth and the fact that some women will not be able to have a 'normal' birth but will need medical interventions. Furthermore, Darra (2009, p. 303) argues that midwives and birth workers need to move away from trying to define and aim for 'normal' birth and instead focus on "being with women, metaphorically holding them," regardless of the type of birth that unfolds.

What then made women feel good in relation to labor/birth? It made women feel good to be treated as important persons—to be listened to, to be informed, to be included and to be cared for. Women spoke about the importance of friendly conversations, kind words, verbal reassurances and guidance about how to handle contractions and traverse the pushing phase. Being greeted and acknowledged with a smile made women feel good. It made women feel good to be supported in concrete body-to-body ways—being held, stroked, comforted, touched and massaged. It made women feel good to be treated as active participants in the birth process and to be informed and included, even if they were having a caesarean section. It made women feel good to be assured of safety. This included both ontological and emotional safety in terms of feeling safe to be, to let go and to negotiate the psychofleshy challenges of labor/birth as well as physical safety—i.e. receiving adequate monitoring and having medical technologies available and implemented when necessary. Being treated with friendliness, warmth and care thus made women feel good during labor/birth. The feelings women have about birth matter and tell us about the power relations circulating with/in particular birth assemblages.

What matters? Sociomaterialities

While heterogeneous and multivocal, the collective weave of voices also demonstrates the territorializing aspects of particular sociomaterial assemblages. While unpredictable and emergent (i.e. a homebirth could be experienced as distressing and a public sector sector experience could be a 'good birth'), sediments and patterns nonetheless emerged in relation to the 'sticky' affective relations circulating within certain birth assemblages. Thus, homebirths were sociomaterial spaces in which women were more likely to be able to enact embodied agency, a sense of presence and receive affirming body-to-body support from those around them. Being at home and surrounded by familiar, comforting objects made women feel good. Women were free to enact 'loud' forms of corporeality in their home environments without censure—some danced, sang, grunted, groaned, shouted and laughed. In homebirth assemblages, women were often surrounded by a multiplicity of supportive bodies and labor/birth became "like a party" (Maggie) or social celebration. At home, women were usually the center of the birth process and were surrounded by a hub of attentive others. This was even the case for the impoverished Jasmine who had an unplanned homebirth with no birth attendant. Birth at home often became an intercorporeal experience in which boundaries between bodies melted away (see Lizette). In these settings, the power of biomedical discourses and frames were muted and diffracted (but not missing). Clockwork scripts continued to infiltrate labor/birth in home spaces (see Chapter 3). However, away from strict hierarchical relations and rules, material-discursive arrangements of biomedical space and equipment, clockwork narratives and biomedical measurements were open to new enactments that enabled sensemaking, embodied agency and body–self connectivity.

The materialization of birth in particular assemblages was also intimately entangled with socioeconomic relations. As argued in Chapters 3 and 4, biomedical practices, norms and material–discursive relations were diffracted in/through socio-economics to result in different articulations of 'risk' and biomedical scripts in particular settings. Instead of being structured along lines of need and an ethics of embodied care, medical interventions, expertise and risk-management practices circulated along lines of profit and privilege. As a result, many low-income women were left *feeling unsafe* during labor/birth because of lack of monitoring and surveillance medicine. At the same time, some privileged women were 'gently coerced' (see Chapter 5) into technological interventions without any coherent rationale/need. The sociomaterial logic/s of birth assemblages in the South African setting thus continue to operate along unacceptable (racialized and classed) bioeconomic lines, resulting in very real 'embodied inequalities' (Spangler, 2011) as some birthing bodies are invisibilized (see Chapter 4), framed as disposable and disregarded, and other bodies are overly visibilized, framed as biomedically risky and subject to unnecessary interventions.

Sociomaterial relations thus clearly *matter* in relation to labor/birth. While not directly articulated or named by women, I have shown in previous chapters how economic and structural relations of power shaped birth assemblages in powerful ways. This often resulted in qualitatively different labor/birth experiences for women across class/race divides. Socioeconomic relations were thus not just abstract, free-floating phenomena but were lived, enacted and embodied in everyday assemblages structured along lines of privilege and marginalization. They were vitalized and enacted in/through scripts and storylines that produced poor, pregnant women as 'guilty bodies,' affective circuits of shaming and the material arrangements of space and objects (see Chapter 5). Sociomaterial relations were thus inextricably entangled with/in birth violations and the production of 'embodied oppressions' (see Chapter 5) during labor/birth.

What matters? Bodies that birth

The collective weave of voices show that birthing bodies are central to what matters to women in relation to birth. The different enactments of the body that births, shaped by ontological frames, affective violences or affirmations and sociomaterial relations, have important implications for the ways women feel about their birth experiences. Women did not articulate a singular, static or homogenous 'birthing body'—instead, birthing bodies were always situated within relational webs and materialized as emergent products of particular assemblages. There was thus no physiological body separate or *apart* from affective, sociosymbolic and material relations of power. Thus, while fleshy physiology did emerge as a powerful agentic force during labor/birth in many stories (see Michelle), it was always part of a wider entanglement of affective, corporeal and sociomaterial relations. The fleshy intensities of labor/birth acted as powerful forces that women had to negotiate and navigate as embodied selves. For many women, the ability to enact forms of body–self connectivity or 'embodied agency' depended on being situated within affirming relational environments that helped to articulate a sense of connection between the forceful contracting or pushing body and the embodied self (see Akrich & Pasveer, 2004). Women needed embodied support, assistance and mediation to read and negotiate fleshy corporeality and articulate forms of embodied agency. Unfortunately, the fleshy vitality of birthing corporeality was often not supported, encouraged or enabled but became the target of disciplining forces and norms geared towards muting and diminishment. As a result, many women spoke of having their efforts to enact embodied agency by moving around freely, enacting different bodily positions, shouting or groaning or doing what felt comfortable, punished or disallowed.

When thinking about what makes women feel good in relation to birth, it is clear that *bodies matter*. Despite sociomaterial differences, most women wanted the following in relation to birth—namely: embodied agency and presence, ontological and physical safety, dignity and embodied care. What matters in relation to birth (from women's perspectives), thus fundamentally involves corporeality and embodied relations. While Lyerly (2006) argues that 'good births' are characterized by three ingredients, namely: agency, dignity and connectedness, she does not go far enough in recognizing the fundamentally embodied aspects of all of these phenomena. 'Agency' in relation to labor/birth is never disembodied or the attribute of an individualist self. Instead, my argument is that 'agency' must always be acknowledged as centrally about embodied agency—i.e. the ability to move and enact forms of corporeality that enable a sense of bodily power and body–self connectivity. Embodied agency is not 'power over' the fleshy process of labor/birth but is fundamentally about a sense of presence and involvement. Many women articulated that being present *with* the psychofleshy process of labor/delivery (whatever that process entailed) by knowing what was happening, being supported, affirmed and recognized and being the central participant of the birth experience, was central to their feelings about birth. On the other side, distressing births were often marked by a sense of disconnection and/or embodied or emotional *absence* in which women felt like they were not active participants or fully present with/in the birth experience.

'Good births' are also fundamentally about a sense of embodied safety (missing from Lyerly's grid). Safety had two key aspects—ontological safety and physical safety. Feeling ontologically safe was about having the bodily freedom to be vulnerable, messy, loud and exposed without being reprimanded or shamed by others. Feel physically safe meant a sense of security that medical technologies were available and that the process of labor/birth was being monitored and in 'safe hands.' As we saw in Chapter 4, 'dignity' was a major concern for women in relation to labor/birth and is outlined as a key ingredient of a 'good birth' by Lyerly (2006). The weave of voices shows that dignity was always an embodied and relational phenomenon, closely tied to the treatment and framing of the corporeal body during labor/birth within particular assemblages. Thus, in homebirth assemblages, the meanings circulating around 'mess' and 'blood and guts' were different to those in medicalized spaces. For example, instead of materializing as threatening, shameful and monstrous, the 'mess' of birthing becomes everyday in Yolande's telling of homebirth (see page 187). Thus, while she acknowledges that birth is "not very dignified" and entails a lot of "messing," with/in this relational matrix, mess and 'blood and guts' *become* a normal and even humorous part of the birth process. Relational and intercorporeal assemblages are thus central to the materialization of 'good births.' Bodily agency, safety and dignity materialized as central features of what made women feel good about their births. These are not 'factors' or 'things' but embodied relations. In addition to embodied agency, safety and dignity, embodied care was also central to what mattered to women during labor/birth. 'Care' is not an abstract principle, ideal or technical checklist but is a fundamentally relational and embodied phenomenon (see Hamington, 2004). It is fleshy, intercorporeal and body-to-body. During labor/birth women want and need embodied care—treatment and touch by gentle, caring and respectful hands (see Angela, Sarayda, Yolande and Lizette). Birth is a challenging psychofleshy experience in which women struggle with body, meaning, self, life/death and the profundity of *giving birth* to new life (Adams, 1994; Lupton & Schmied, 2013). As a result, the provision of care during labor/birth requires an orientation towards embodied care—caring with bodies, words, hands, gestures, smiles, flesh and touch.

The relational, material-discursive and affective matrix of labor/birth thus shapes women's feelings about birth and their corporeal selves. Birthing bodies are open and permeable to the affective and bodily energies transfused in/through birth assemblages. Women feel good when they are treated with respect, positive affirmations, embodied dignity and body-to-body care. The feelings women have about birth matter and tell us about the sociomaterial, corporeal and ontological power relations framing birth in particular assemblages. Moreover, the ways in which birthing bodies are treated reveal fundamental 'truths' about societal attitudes towards women. While 'women' are not one category and differences abound according to intersecting social relations of marginalization/privilege, the fleshy process of labor/birth always engenders corporeal vulnerability in which women are dependent on others for embodied care, support and assistance. Women can be affirmed or diminished by the ways in which they are treated (by others, institutions and sociomaterial structures) during labor/birth.

Vitalizing birth politics requires putting corporeality at the center of what matters in relation to birth. Across race–class divides women want to be able to enact embodied agency and presence, feel safe (physically and ontologically), maintain dignity and be given 'embodied care' (Hamington, 2004) from those around them. Working towards the realization of 'good births' for all women thus necessitates the development of an embodied ethics of birth that respects the corporeal birth process, enables embodied agency and presence, ensures ontological and physical safety, affirms dignity and provides body-to-body affirmative care. The development of such an embodied ethics requires the creation of alternative ontologies of birthing bodies rooted in women's own fleshy articulations of what matters in relation to birth.

8

CLOSING

This book has explored the corporeal politics of birth. Using women's birth narratives as openings, I explored the ways in which material-discursive frames and sociomaterial power relations were enacted, consolidated, negotiated and resisted in everyday acts of telling. In the South African context, birth was shown to be indelibly shaped by racialized patriarchy, socioeconomic marginalization/s and a bifurcated health system. However, at the level of everyday enactments, the private and public 'sectors' in South Africa are not fixed categories of difference but comprised of multiple birth assemblages. Biomedical power was shown to operate in/ through all of these spaces in diffractive ways, colliding with other modes of socio- materiality. As a result, I argued that biomedical power is radically heterogeneous and can materialize as constraining, oppressive, enabling and/or empowering in different situations. There is no 'natural' birth (as pure instinct or physiology) that stands separate and *apart* from sociomaterial relations and there is no birthing body that materializes separately and independently from sociomaterial contexts, histori- cal relations and sociosymbolic discursive frames and ontologies.

Bodies that birth showed that biomedical vocabularies were integral to the con- struction of (ambiguous) modes of birthing agency and stories about birth (see particularly Chapters 3 and 4). Biomedical frames, storylines (i.e. the clockwork narrative), technologies and practices were, however, not equally available to all women. Low-income women often struggled to gain access to biomedical services and to the 'clockwork narrative.' They were often refused information about their own labors that might have helped them to manage and cope with their labor/ birth experiences. Biomedical power thus intra-acted with other modes of power and marginalization to make certain birthing bodies invisible and rendered them unworthy of medical care. As a form of hierarchical knowledge, ontological 'truth' and sociomaterial practices, biomedicalized birth collided with racialized, classed and gendered power relations to produce public sector birth assemblages often marked by mistreatment, dignity violations, embodied oppression/s and poor quality of care. In the private sector, birth 'choices' and agency are ostensibly promised to pregnant women but collisions between neoliberal bioeconomics, patriarchal obstetrics, morally infused risk discourses and intensive forms of obstetric technocracy resulted in situations where women often had no real 'choices' available to them during labor/birth (see Chapter 5).

Birth politics emerged as fraught in the South African context. Some women give birth in well-resourced and safe homes with private midwives, doulas, birthing pools and toys, supportive partners and the full range of domestic comforts (i.e. warmth, food, furniture, baby, birthing and mothering supplies), while other women give birth in community clinics situated in the midst of neighborhoods racked by gang warfare, the sounds of gun fire and high rates of violence. In these low-resourced clinics, some women labor without food, water, blankets, pillows or any support from health care providers. Some of these poor women experience non-interventionist, so-called 'natural' births in which they are alone, invisible and receive little to no medical attention in clinic settings while others experience highly medicalized births (i.e. with inductions, rupturing of membranes, immobilization via EFM's and intravenous drips and episiotomies) in public hospitals. In our conversations, some low-income women resisted birthing injustices and narrated bold testimonies of violation while others were passively accepting and regarded local cultures of birth (including mistreatment) as 'normal.' Unlike women who planned homebirths, some privileged and well-resourced South African women are not interested in birth as life event or 'experience' and choose to be delivered surgically by elective caesarean section. These births unfolded in surgical theatres surrounded by clinical equipment, sterilized tools and highly trained obstetric experts outfitted in surgical garb. Women in South Africa thus experience a wide range of possible births and their degree of happiness and 'satisfaction' with their birth experiences is not always predictable.

As argued in this book, the use of medical technologies and interventions does not always equal unhappiness and a 'natural' or vaginal birth does not always equal satisfaction and contentment. Furthermore, the meanings of what is 'natural' or 'normal' in relation to birth are slippery. In *Bodies that Birth*, I have explored a wide range of birth narratives—from stories of elective caesareans to homebirths (planned and unplanned), disappointing births, enjoyable births and births marked by violation. The birthing bodies reproduced in women's narratives were complex, multiple and emergent sociomaterialities. In these stories, birthing bodies emerged as *different entities* as a result of the diffractive play of intra-acting sociomaterial forces, frames and norms. They were *inscribed* by biomedical vocabularies, racialized ideologies and socioeconomics (see Chapter 3), *disciplined* by risk and moral imperatives (see Chapter 4), *shaped* by 'gentle violence' and *violated* through/by affective and embodied violence (see Chapter 5). At the same time, birthing bodies were also shown to be embodied capacities with the power to become 'loud' and resistant or 'speak back' against injustices (see Chapter 6). Thus, while birth was always thoroughly embodied, the birthing body was never one. Birthing bodies resisted singular interpretations.

This book highlighted the ontological politics (Mol, 2002) of birth. Ontological framings of birthing bodies (see Chapter 2) have diffractive, socioaffective and material effects that shape the ways women are treated during labor/birth. As a result, it *matters* what frames we use to think about birthing bodies. Frames are not just abstract, free-floating phenomenon but sociomaterialities that vitalize and shape birth (and birthing bodies) in particular ways. This is 'ontological politics' (Mol, 2002). In relation to birth, ontological politics means recognizing that frames are an intra-acting component of birth assemblages and materialize in/as everyday material-discursive enactments of birth. As argued in Chapter 2, biomedical ontologies reproduce body/mind dualism and frame/enact the birthing body as a physiological or natural object apart from embodied personhood. This was shown to have powerful affective and relational consequences within birth assemblages as women were routinely treated as depersonalized body-objects (*Körper*) and subjected to embodied oppressions vitalized by biomedical ontologies of birthing bodies (see Chapter 5). Phallocentric ontological frames were also shown *becoming* with/in women's own expectations, fears and imaginings about labor/birth (see Chapter 4). As a result, framings of laboring/birthing bodies as disgusting, monstrous and abject circulated within women's stories and shaped the choices that they made about birth and their feelings about their female corporeality. Of course, ontologies of birthing bodies were never coherently univocal or discrete but always entangled with/in and diffracted through other frames and power relations. As a result, black and poor pregnant bodies were enacted as particularly disgusting, abhorrent and undeserving of medical treatment via the diffractive, intra-acting frames of biomedicine, racialized patriarchy and socioeconomics. Framing/s of birthing bodies as risky and as passive body-objects were also shown to *affect* women's experiences of labor/birth, resulting in enactments of hesitant embodiment, lack of confidence and the loss of bodily agency (see Chapter 5).

As explored in Chapter 5, violations during labor/birth often targeted the power and vitality of fleshy laboring/birthing bodies, working to erase, mute and constrict women's capacities to enact forms of embodied agency during labor/birth. As a result, many women were subjected to forms of 'embodied oppression' that worked to deny their embodied personhood, agency and rights to bodily privacy and dignity during birth. Birthing bodies thus emerged as central to relations of power, ontological politics and violations. Birthing bodies were framed in multiple directions, caught in an entangled matrix of sociomaterial relations, subject to both gentle and overt violence, invisiblized, hypervisibilized and disciplined both from the outside and the inside. At the same time, bodies spoke back and enacted forms of resistance in/through narratives. As a result, birthing bodies emerged in women's stories as agentic and powerful capacities, laughing, subverting, exceeding and 'talking back' against erasure. The psychofleshy complexities of labor/birth and the embodied perspective of the birthgiver (whether pleasurable or distressing) were enacted in/through fleshy and excessive tellings. Normative ontologies that inscribe laboring/birthing bodies as passive objects or as separable from embodied personhood were thus both reiterated and disrupted in women's stories. Ontological frames were central forces vitalizing and shaping material-discursive practices and the treatment of laboring/birthing bodies. They were also sticky with affects and central to women's feelings about their labor/birth experiences.

In *Bodies that Birth* I have argued that there is no singular birthing body standing apart and separate from politics, power and sociomateriality. Fundamentally, birthing bodies *matter*—to politics, to birthing women and in efforts to reimagine birth as embodied ethicality. Putting bodies at the center of analysis has the potential to vitalize the politics of birth, opening new lines of thinking for the development of activisms and interventions to improve women's birth experiences. While activisms, analyses and interventions remain stuck within dualist and polarizing frames of birthing bodies (see Chapter 2) we will not be able to hear what women are saying matters to them in relation to birth. Taking women's voices seriously means recognizing the importance of the relational, embodied and affective contexts in which birthgiving occurs (see Chapter 7). The project of vitalizing birth politics requires the development of alternative ontologies of birth that valorize embodied ethics and privilege the embodied personhood of birthgivers. Until we recognize the everyday material implications of the frames we use to think about birthing bodies, there will be no possibility for the vitalization of birth politics or the improvement of maternity services. Birth is a complex entanglement of affective, ontological, sociomaterial and embodied politics. To move beyond stagnant debates, we need to frame labor/birth as embodied ethicality, involving a psycho-fleshy, emotional and vulnerable corporeality deeply affected and interpenetrated by relational flows, affective violence and sociomaterial structures. Vitalizing birth politics means developing ethico-ontological frames that recognize birthgivers as embodied persons situated within a mesh of corpomaterial relations. It also means developing ontologies that *value birth* and birthgivers. Finally, the realization of 'good births' for all women requires active intersectional social justice work to counter and challenge the increasing bioeconomic logic of maternity services and social relations of power that continue to marginalize persons on the basis of socio-economics, race and other markers of bodily difference.

REFERENCES

Acker, M. (2009). Breast is best . . . but not everywhere: Ambivalent sexism and attitudes towards private and public breastfeeding. *Sex Roles, 61* (7), 476–490.

Adair, V. (2002). Branded with infamy: Inscriptions of poverty and class in the United States. *Signs, 27* (2), 451–471.

Adams, A. (1994). *Reproducing the womb: Images of childbirth in science, feminist theory, and literature.* Ithaca: Cornell University Press.

Ahmed, S. (2014). *The cultural politics of emotion.* Edinburgh: Edinburgh University Press.

Akrich, M. and Pasveer, B. (2004). Embodiment and disembodiment in childbirth narratives. *Body and Society, 10* (2–3), 63–83.

Alaimo, S. (2010). *Bodily natures: Science, environment and the bodily self.* Bloomington: Indiana University Press.

Alaimo, S. and Hekman, S. (2008). (Eds.). *Material feminisms.* Bloomington: Indiana University Press.

Annandale, E. and Clark, J. (1996). What is gender? Feminist theory and the sociology of human reproduction. *Sociology of Health and Illness, 18* (1), 17–44.

Arms, S. (1977). *Immaculate deception: A new look at women and childbirth in America.* New York: Bantham Books (original work published in 1975).

Armstrong, D. (1995). The rise of surveillance medicine. *Sociology of Health and Illness, 17* (3), 393–404.

Arney, W. (1982). *Power and the profession of obstetrics.* Chicago: University of Chicago Press.

Ashmore, M., MacMillan, K. and Brown, S. (2004). It's a scream: Professional hearing and tape fetishism. *Journal of Pragmatics, 36* (2), 349–374.

Ayers, S. and Pickering, A. (2005). Women's expectations and experiences of birth. *Psychology and Health, 20* (1), 79–92.

Ayob, R. (2014). An observation of the caesarean section rate at a teaching hospital in Johannesburg. Unpublished Masters dissertation, University of the Witwatersrand.

Baker, S., Choi, P. and Henshaw, C. (2005). 'I felt as though I'd been in jail': Women's experiences of maternity care during labor, delivery, and the immediate postpartum. *Feminism and Psychology, 15* (3), 315–342.

Balsam, R. (2012). *Women's bodies in psychoanalysis.* New York: Routledge.

Barad, K. (2007). *Meeting the universe halfway: Quantam physics and the entanglement of matter and meaning*. Durham: Duke University Press.

Bartky, S. (1990). *Femininity and domination: Studies in the phenomenology of oppression*. New York: Routledge.

Bartlett, A. (2002). Breastfeeding as headwork: Corporeal feminism and meanings for breastfeeding. *Women's Studies International Forum, 25* (3), 373–382.

Bateman, C. (2014). Dismal obs/gynae training contributing to maternal deaths— Motsoaledi. *South African Medical Journal, 104* (10), 656–657.

Battersby, C. (1998). *The phenomenal woman: Feminist metaphysics and the patterns of identity*. Cambridge: Polity Press.

Beck, C. (2004). Birth trauma: In the eye of the beholder. *Nursing Research, 53* (1), 28–35.

Beck, C. (2009). Traumatic birth and its sequelae. *Journal of Trauma and Dissociation*, 10(2), 189–203.

Beckett, K. (2005). Choosing cesarean: Feminism and the politics of childbirth in the United States. *Feminist Theory, 6* (3), 251–275.

Behruzi, R., Hatem, M., Fraser, W., Goulet, L.M. and Misago, C. (2010). Facilitators and barriers in the humanization of childbirth practice in Japan. *BMC Pregnancy and Childbirth, 10* (25). https://doi.org/10.1186/1471-2393-10-25.

Bennett, J. (2010). *Vibrant matter: An ecology of things*. Durham: Duke University Press.

Betterton, R. (2006). Promising monsters: Pregnant bodies, artistic subjectivity, and maternal imagination. *Hypatia, 21* (1), 80–100.

Blauuw, D. and Penn-Kekana, L. (2010). Maternal health. *South African Health Review*, 3–28. www.popline.org/node/229536

Blommaert, J. (2006). Applied ethnopoetics. *Narrative Inquiry, 16* (1), 181–190.

Blum, L. (1999). *At the breast: Ideologies of breastfeeding and motherhood in contemporary United States*. Boston: Beacon Press.

Boden, G. (2015). Childbirth as entertainment. *AIMS Journal, 24* (4). www.aims.org. uk/?Journal/Vol24No4/birthAsEntertainment.htm

Bohren, M.A., Vogel, J.P., Hunter, E.C., Lutsiv, O., Makh, S.K., Souza, J.P. . . . Gülmezoglu, A.M. (2015). The mistreatment of women during childbirth in health facilities globally: A mixed-methods systematic review. *PLoS Medicine, 12* (6), e1001847.

Bohren, M.A., Vogel, J.P., Tunçalp, Ö., Fawole, B., Titiloye, M.A., Olutayo, A.O. . . . Hindin, M. (2016). 'By slapping their laps, the patients will know that you truly care for her': A qualitative study on social norms and acceptability of the mistreatment of women during childbirth in Abuja, Nigeria. *SSM Population Health, 2*, 640–655.

Boulous-Walker, M. (1998). *Philosophy and the maternal body: Reading silence*. London: Routledge.

Bourdieu, P. (2001). *Masculine domination*. Stanford: Stanford University Press.

Boyer, K. (2011). 'The way to break the taboo is to do the taboo thing': Breastfeeding in public and citizen-activism in the UK. *Health and Place, 17* (2), 430–437.

Boyer, K. (2012). Affect, corporeality, and the limits of belonging: Breastfeeding in public in the contemporary UK. *Health and Place, 18* (3), 552–560.

Bradby, B. (1998). Like a video: The sexualization of childbirth in Bolivia. *Reproductive Health Matters, 6* (12), 50–56.

Bradshaw, D. and Dorrington, R. (2012). Maternal mortality ratio: Trends in the vital registration data. *South African Journal of Obstetrics and Gynaeology, 18*, 38–42.

Bradshaw, D., Dorrington, R. and Laubsher, R. (2012). *Rapid mortality surveillance report 2011*. Cape Town, South Africa: South African Medical Research Council.

Braidotti, R. (2013). *The posthuman*. Cambridge: Polity Press.

Breen, D. (1975). *The birth of a first child*. London: Tavistock.

Bridges, K. (2011). *Reproducing race: An ethnography of pregnancy as a site of racialization*. Berkeley: University of California Press.

Brubaker, S. (2007). Denied, embracing, and resisting medicalization: African American teen mothers' perceptions of formal pregnancy and childbirth care. *Gender and Society*, *21* (4), 528–552.

Bruner, J. (1987). Life as narrative. *Social Research*, *54* (1), 11–32.

Burr, V. (2015). *Social constructionism*. London: Routledge.

Butler, J. (1993). *Bodies that matter: On the discursive limits of sex*. New York: Routledge.

Butler, J. (2016). *Frames of war: When is life grievable?* London: Verso (original work published 2009).

Cahill, H. (2001). Male appropriation and medicalization of childbirth: An historical analysis. *Journal of Advanced Nursing*, *33* (3), 334–342.

Carter, S. (2009). Gender performances during labor and birth in the midwives model of care. *Gender Issues*, *26*, 205–223.

Carter, S. (2010). Beyond control: Body and self in women's childbearing narratives. *Sociology of Health and Illness*, *32* (7), 993–1009.

Casper, M. and Moore, L. (2009). *Missing bodies: The politics of visibility*. New York: New York University Press.

Chadwick, R. (2009). Between bodies, cultural scripts and power: The reproduction of birthing subjectivities in homebirth narratives. *Subjectivity*, *27*, 109–133.

Chadwick, R. (2012). Fleshy enough? Notes towards embodied analysis in critical qualitative research. *Gay and Lesbian Issues and Psychology Review*, *8* (2), 82–97.

Chadwick, R. (2014). Bodies talk: On the challenges of hearing childbirth counter-stories. In S. McKenzie-Mohr and M. Lafrance (Eds.), *Women voicing resistance: Discursive and narrative explorations* (pp. 44–63). London: Routledge.

Chadwick, R. (2016). Obstetric violence in South Africa. *South African Medical Journal*, *106* (1), 1–2.

Chadwick, R. (2017a) Embodied methodologies: Challenges, reflections and strategies. *Qualitative Research*, *17* (1), 54–74.

Chadwick, R. (2017b). Ambiguous subjects: Obstetric violence, assemblage and South African birth narratives. *Feminism and Psychology*, *27* (4), 489–509.

Chadwick, R. and Foster, D. (2013). Technologies of gender and childbirth choices: Homebirth, elective caesarean and white femininities in South Africa. *Feminism and Psychology*, *23* (3), 317–338.

Chadwick, R. and Foster, D. (2014). Negotiating risky bodies: Childbirth and constructions of risk. *Health, Risk and Society*, *16* (1), 68–83.

Chadwick, R., Cooper, D. and Harries, J. (2014). Narratives of distress about birth in South African public sector settings: A qualitative study. *Midwifery*, *30*, 862–868.

Chertok, L. (1969). *Motherhood and personality: Psychosomatic aspects of childbirth*. London: Tavistock.

Chesler, P. (1979). *With child: A diary of motherhood*. New York: Thomas Y. Crowell Publishers.

Cheyney, M. (2008). Homebirth as systems-challenging praxis: Knowledge, power, and intimacy in the birthplace. *Qualitative Health Research*, *18* (2), 254–267.

Christiaens, W. and Bracke, P. (2009). Place of birth and satisfaction with childbirth in Belgium and the Netherlands. *Midwifery*, *25* (2), e11–e19.

Cindoglu, D. and Sayan-Cengiz, F. (2010). Medicalization discourse and modernity: Contested meanings over childbirth in contemporary Turkey. *Health Care for Women International*, *31* (3), 221–243.

Colaguori, C. (2010). Symbolic violence and the violation of human rights: Continuing the sociological critique of domination. *International Journal of Criminology and Sociological Theory*, *3* (2), 388–400.

Collins, P. and Bilge, S. (2016). *Intersectionality*. Cambridge: Polity Press.

Coole, D. and Frost, S. (2010). (Eds.). *New materialisms: Ontology, agency, and politics*. Durham: Duke University Press.

Cosslett, T. (1994). *Women writing childbirth: Modern discourses of motherhood*. Manchester: Manchester University Press.

Coxon, K., Sandall, J. and Fulop, N. (2014) To what extent are women free to choose where to give birth? How discourses of risk, blame and responsibility influence birth place decisions. *Health, Risk and Society*, *16* (1), 51–67.

Creedy, D., Shochet, I. and Horsfall, J. (2000). Childbirth and the development of acute trauma symptoms: Incidence and contributing factors. *Birth*, *27* (2), 104–111.

Crossley, M. (2007). Childbirth, complications, and the illusion of 'choice': A case study. *Feminism and Psychology*, *17* (4), 543–563.

Crossley, N. (1996). Body-subject/body-power: Agency, inscription and control in Foucault and Merleau-Ponty. *Body and Society*, *1* (2), 99–116.

Cusk, R. (2001). *A life's work: On becoming a mother*. London: Fourth Estate.

D'Ambruoso, L., Abbey, M. and Hussein, J. (2005). Please understand when I cry out in pain: Women's accounts of maternity services during labor and delivery in Ghana. *BMC Public Health*, *5*, 140.

Darra, S. (2009). 'Normal', 'natural', 'good' or 'good-enough' birth: Examining the concepts. *Nursing Inquiry*, *16* (4), 297–305.

Davis, D. and Walker, K. (2010a). Re-discovering the maternal body in midwifery through an exploration of theories of embodiment. *Midwifery*, *26*, 457–462.

Davis, D. and Walker, K. (2010b). The corporeal, the social and space/place: Exploring intersections from a midwifery perspective in New Zealand. *Gender, Place and Culture*, *17* (3), 377–391.

Davis, D. and Walker, K. (2013). Towards an 'optics of power': Technologies of surveillance and discipline and case-loading midwifery practice in New Zealand. *Gender, Place and Culture*, *20* (5), 597–612.

Davis-Floyd, R. (1994). The technocratic body: American childbirth as cultural expression. *Social Science and Medicine*, *38* (8), 1125–1140.

Davis-Floyd, R. (2001). The technocratic, humanistic, and holistic paradigms of childbirth. *International Journal of Gynecology and Obstetrics*, *75* (1), 5–23.

Davis-Floyd, R. (2003). *Birth as an American rite of passage*. Berkeley: University of California Press (original work published 1992).

DeLanda, M. (2006). *A new philosophy of society: Assemblage theory and social complexity*. London: Continuum.

Deleuze, G. and Guattari, F. (1987). *A thousand plateaus: Capitalism and schizophrenia*. Minnesota: University of Minnesota Press.

Deleuze, G. and Parnet, C. (1987). *Dialogues*. Columbia: Columbia University Press.

Deutsch, H. (1944). *The psychology of women: A psychoanalytic interpretation, Volumes 1 and 2*. New York: Grune & Stratton.

Diamond, I. (1994). *Fertile ground: Women, earth, and the limits of control*. Boston: Beacon Press.

Diaz-Tello, F. (2016). Invisible wounds: Obstetric violence in the United States. *Reproductive Health Matters*, *24*, 56–64.

Dick-Read. G. (1933). *Natural childbirth*. London: Heinemann.

Dick-Read, G. (1963). *Childbirth without fear: The principles and practice of natural childbirth.* London: Heinemann (original work published 1942).

Dillaway, H. and Brubaker, S. (2006). Intersectionality and childbirth: How women from different social locations discuss epidural use. *Race, Gender and Class, 13,* 16–41.

Dixon, L. (2015). Obstetrics in a time of violence: Mexican midwives critique routine hospital practices. *Medical Anthropology Quarterly, 29* (4), 437–454.

Doering, S., Entwisle. D. and Quinlan, D. (1980). Modeling the quality of women's birth experiences. *Journal of Health and Social Behavior, 21,* 12–21.

Dolezal, L. (2015). *The body and shame: Phenomenology, feminism, and the socially shaped body.* Lanham: Lexington Books.

D'Oliveira, A., Diniz, S. and Schraibe, L. (2002). Violence against women in healthcare institutions: An emerging problem. *Lancet, 359* (9318), 1681–1685.

Durik, A., Shibley Hyde, J. and Clark, R. (2000). Sequelae of cesarean and vaginal deliveries: Psychosocial outcomes for mothers and infants. *Developmental Psychology, 36* (2), 251–260.

Dzomeki, M. (2011). Maternal satisfaction with care during labor: A case study of the Mampong-Ashanti district hospital maternity unit in Ghana. *International Journal of Nursing and Midwifery, 3* (3), 30–34.

Earle, S. (2003). 'Bumps and boobs': Fatness and women's experiences of pregnancy. *Women's Studies International Forum, 26* (3), 245–252.

Ebert, T. (1996). *Ludic feminism and after: Postmodernism, desire, and labor in late capitalism.* Ann Arbor: The University of Michigan Press.

Econex. (2013). The South African private healthcare sector: Role and contribution to the economy. *Research Note,* 32. Accessed 23 July 2017. https://econex.co.za/wp-content/uploads/2015/03/econex_researchnote_32.pdf

Edwards, N. and Murphy-Lawless, J. (2006). The instability of risk: Women's perspectives on risk and safety in childbirth. In A. Symon (Ed.), *Risk and choice in maternity care: An international perspective* (pp. 35–50). Philadelphia: Elsevier/Churchill Livingstone.

Einstein, G. and Shildrick, M. (2009). The postconventional body: Retheorising women's health. *Social Science and Medicine, 69,* 293–300.

Elmir, R., Schmied, V., Wilkes, L. and Jackson, D. (2010). Women's perceptions and experiences of a traumatic birth: A meta-ethnography. *Journal of Advanced Nursing, 66* (10), 2142–2153.

El-Nemer, A., Downe, S. and Small, N. (2006). 'She would help me from the heart': An ethnography of Egyptian women in labor. *Social Science and Medicine, 62,* 81–92.

Elvey, A. (2003). The material given: Bodies, pregnant bodies, and earth. *Australian Feminist Studies, 18* (41), 199–209.

Ettorre, E. (1998). Re-shaping the space between bodies and culture: Embodying the bio-medicalized body. *Sociology of Health and Illness, 20* (4), 548–555.

Ettorre, E. (2002). *Reproductive genetics, gender, and the body.* London: Routledge.

Faith, K. (1994). Resistance: Lessons from Foucault and feminism. In L. Radtke and H. Stam (Eds.), *Power/gender: Social relations in theory and practice* (pp. 36–66). London: Sage.

Fannin, M. (2003). Domesticating birth in the hospital: 'Family-centred' birth and the emergence of 'homelike' birthing rooms. *Antipode, 35* (3), 513–535.

Fathalla, M. (2006). Human rights aspects of safe motherhood. *Best Practice and Research Clinical Obstetrics and Gynaecology,* 20 (3), 409–419.

Fausto-Sterling, A. (2005). The bare bones of sex: Part 1—Sex and gender. *Signs, 30* (2), 1491–1527.

Feeley, C., Burns, E., Adams, E. and Thomson, G. (2015). Why do some women choose to freebirth? A meta-thematic synthesis, part one. *Evidence Based Midwifery, 13* (1), 4–9.

Forssén, A. (2012). Lifelong significance of disempowering experiences in prenatal and maternity care: Interviews with elderly Swedish women. *Qualitative Health Research*, *22* (11), 1535–1546.

Foucault, M. (1972). *The archeology of knowledge and the discourse on language*. New York: Pantheon Books.

Foucault, M. (1979). *Discipline and punish: The birth of the prison*. Harmondsworth: Penguin Books (original work published 1975).

Foucault, M. (1980). *Power/knowledge: Selected interviews and other writings 1972–1977*. Sussex: The Harvester Press. (Edited by C. Gordon).

Foucault, M. (1984). Truth and method. In P. Rabinow (Ed.), *The Foucault reader* (pp. 31–120). New York: Pantheon.

Foucault, M. (1990). *The history of sexuality: An introduction, volume 1*. New York: Vintage Books (original work published 1976).

Foucault, M. (1997). Technologies of the self. In P. Rabinow (Ed.), *Michel Foucault: Ethics, subjectivity and truth* (pp. 223–251). New York: The New Press.

Fowles, E. (1998). Labor concerns of women two months after delivery. *Birth*, *25* (4), 235–240.

Fox, N. and Alldred, P. (2015). New materialist social enquiry: Designs, methods and the research-assemblage. *International Journal of Social Research Methodology*, *18* (4), 399–414.

Fox, N. and Alldred, P. (2017). *Sociology and the new materialism: Theory, research, action*. Los Angeles: Sage.

Fox, B. and Worts, D. (1999). Revisiting the critique of medicalized childbirth: A contribution to the sociology of birth. *Gender and Society*, *13* (3), 326–346.

Frank, A. (1990). Bringing bodies back in: A decade review. *Theory, Culture and Society*, *7* (1), 131–162.

Frank, A. (1995). *The wounded storyteller: Body, illness and ethics*. Chicago: The University of Chicago Press.

Frank, A. (2005). What is dialogical research and why should we do it? *Qualitative Health Research*, *15* (7), 964–974.

Frank, A. (2010). *Letting stories breathe: A socio-narratology*. Chicago: The University of Chicago Press.

Freedman, L. and Kruk, M. (2014). Disrespect and abuse of women in childbirth: Challenging the global quality and accountability agendas. *Lancet*, *384*, e42–e44.

Freedman, L., Ramsey, K., Abuya, T., Bellows, B., Ndwiga, C., Warren, C. . . . . Mbaruku, G. (2014). Defining disrespect and abuse of women in childbirth: A research, policy, and rights agenda. *Bulletin of World Health Organization*, *92*, 915–917.

Frost, S. (2011). The implications of new materialisms for feminist epistemology. In H. Grasswick (Ed.), *Feminist epistemology and philosophy of science: Power in knowledge* (pp. 69–84). Dordrecht: Springer.

Galtung, J. (1969). Violence, peace, and peace research. *Journal of Peace Research*, *6* (3), 167–191.

Garry, A. (2001). Medicine and medicalization: A response to Purdy. *Bioethics*, *15* (3), 262–269.

Gatens, M. (1996). *Imaginary bodies: Ethics, power and corporeality*. New York: Routledge.

Geerts, E. and van der Tuin, I. (2013). From intersectionality to interference: Feminist onto-epistemological reflections on the politics of experience. *Women's Studies International Forum*, *41*, 171–178.

Ghani, R. and Berggren, V. (2011). Parturient needs during labor: Egyptian women's perspective towards childbirth experience, a step towards excellence in clinical practice. *Journal of Basic and Applied Scientific Research*, *1* (12), 2935–2945.

Gibbons, J. and Thomson, A. (2001). Women's expectations and experiences of childbirth. *Midwifery*, *17*, 302–313.

Gibson, D. (2004). The gaps in the gaze in South African hospitals. *Social Science and Medicine, 59*, 2013–2024.

Gill, R. (2008). Empowerment/sexism: Figuring female sexual agency in contemporary advertising. *Feminism and Psychology, 8* (1), 35–60.

Gill, R. and Scharff, C. (2011). (Eds.). Introduction. In R. Gill and C. Scharff (Eds.), *New Femininities: Postfeminism, neoliberalism and subjectivity* (pp. 1–20). London: Palgrave Macmillan.

Gilligan, C., Spencer, R., Weinberg, K. and Bertsch, K. (2003). On the listening guide: A voice-centred relational method. In P. Camic, J. Rhodes and L. Yardley (Eds.), *Qualitative research in psychology: Expounding perspectives in methodology and design* (pp. 157–172). Washington, DC: American Psychological Association.

Goer, H. (2010). Cruelty in maternity wards: Fifty years later. *The Journal of Perinatal Education, 19* (3), 33–42.

Goldberg, L. (2002). Rethinking the birthing body: Cartesian dualism and perinatal nursing. *Journal of Advanced Nursing, 37*, 5, 446–451.

Goldstein, D. (2003). *Laughter out of place: Race, class, violence, and sexuality in a Rio shanty-town*. Berkeley: University of California Press.

Gordon, A. (1996). *Ghostly matters: Haunting and the sociological imagination*. Minneapolis: University of Minnesota Press.

Gould, D. (2000) Normal labor: A concept analysis. *Journal of Advanced Nursing, 31* (2), 418–427.

Green, J. and Baston, H. (2003). Feeling in control during childbirth: Concepts, correlates and consequences. *Birth, 30* (4), 235–247.

Grosz, E. (1989). *Sexual subversions: Three French feminists*. Sydney: Allen & Unwin.

Grosz, E. (1990). The body of signification. In J. Fletcher and A. Benjamin (Eds.), *Abjection, melancholia and love: The work of Julia Kristeva* (pp. 80–103). London: Routledge.

Grosz, E. (1994). *Volatile bodies: Towards a corporeal feminism*. Bloomington: Indiana University Press.

Hacking, I. (1990). *The taming of chance*. Cambridge: Cambridge University Press.

Hames-Garcia, M. (2008). How real is race? In S. Alaimo and S. Hekman (Eds.), *Material feminisms* (pp. 308–339). Bloomington: Indiana University Press.

Hamington, M. (2004). *Embodied care: Jane Adams, Maurice Merleau-Ponty, and Feminist Ethics*. Urbana: University of Illinois Press.

Hanson, C. (2004). *A cultural history of pregnancy: Pregnancy, medicine and culture, 1750–2000*. Hampshire: Palgrave Macmillan.

Haraway, D. (1992). *Promises of monsters: A regenerative politics for inappropriate/d others*. New York: Routledge.

Haraway, D. (1997). *Modest witness @ second millennium. Female-man meets onco-mouse: Feminism and technoscience*. New York: Routledge.

Haraway, D. (2016). *Staying with the trouble: Making kin in the Chthulucene*. Durham: Duke University Press.

Hardt, M. and Negri, A. (2000). *Empire*. Cambridge, MA: Harvard University Press.

Haslanger, S. (2012). *Resisting reality: Social constructionism and social critique*. Oxford: Oxford University Press.

Hausman, B. (2007). Things (not) to do with breasts in public: Maternal embodiment and the biocultural politics of infant feeding. *New Literary History, 38* (3), 479–504.

Haydock, S. (2014). *Unhindered childbirth: Wisdom for the passage of unassisted birth*. CreateSpace Independent Publishing Platform.

Hekman, S. (2010). *The material of knowledge: Feminist disclosures*. Bloomington: Indiana University Press.

Helen, I. (2004). Technics over life: Risk, ethics and the existential condition in high-tech antenatal care. *Economy and Society, 33* (1), 28–51.

Hennessey, R. (1993). *Materialist feminism and the politics of discourse.* New York: Routledge.

Henriques, J., Hollway, W., Urwin, C., Venn, C. and Walkerdine, V. (1998). *Changing the subject: Psychology, social regulation and subjectivity.* London: Routledge (original work published 1984).

Hoberman, J. (2005). The primitive pelvis: The role of racial folklore in obstetrics and gynaeology during the twentieth century. In C. Forth and I. Crozier (Eds.), *Body parts: Critical explorations in corporeality* (pp. 85–104). Lanham: Lexington Books.

Hodnett, E. (2002). Pain and women's satisfaction with the experience of childbirth: A systematic review. *American Journal of Obstetrics and Gynecology, 186,* 160–172.

Hofberg, K. and Brockington, I. (2000). Tokophobia: An unreasoning dread of childbirth. *British Journal of Psychiatry, 176,* 83–85.

Hollway, W. (2015). *Knowing mothers: Researching maternal identity change.* Basingstoke: Palgrave Macmillan.

Humphreys, K. (1998). Medicalized maternity: An investigation into women's experiences of medicalized childbirth. Unpublished Masters dissertation, University of Cape Town.

Jacobson, N. (2007). Dignity and health: A review. *Social Science and Medicine, 64* (2), 292–302.

Janssen, P., Carty, E. and Reime, B. (2006). Satisfaction with planned place of birth among midwifery clients in British Columbia. *Journal of Midwifery and Women's Health, 51* (2), 91–97.

Jasen, P. (1997). Race, culture and the colonization of childbirth in Northern Canada. *Social History of Medicine, 10* (3), 383–400.

Jewkes, R. and Penn-Kekana, L. (2015). Mistreatment of women in childbirth: Time for action on this important dimension of violence against women. *PLoS Medicine, 12,* e1001849.

Jewkes, R., Abrahams, N. and Mvo, Z. (1998). Why do nurses abuse patients? Reflections from South African obstetric services. *Social Science and Medicine, 47* (11), 1781–1795.

Johnson, C. (2016). *Maternal transition: A North–South politics of pregnancy and childbirth.* New York: Routledge (original work published 2014).

Jordan, B. (1993). *Birth in four cultures: A cross-cultural investigation of childbirth in Yucatan, Holland, Sweden, and the United States.* Illinois: Waveland Press (original work published 1978).

Keeton, C. (2010). The death of the natural birth? *Sunday Times,* 21 March 2010.

Khalil, D. (2009). Nurses' attitudes towards 'difficult' and 'good' patients in eight public hospitals. *International Journal of Nursing Practice, 15,* 437–443.

Khosla, R., Zampas, C., Vogel, J., Bohren, M., Roseman, M. and Erdman, J. (2016). International human rights and the mistreatment of women during childbirth. *Health and Human Rights, 18* (2), 131–143.

Kitzinger, S. (1992). Birth and violence against women: Generating hypotheses from women's accounts of unhappiness after childbirth. In H. Roberts. (Ed.), *Women's health matters* (pp. 63–80). London: Routledge.

Klassen, P. (2001). *Blessed events: Religion and homebirth in America.* Princeton: Princeton University Press.

Kornelsen, J. (2005). Essences and imperatives: An investigation of technology in childbirth. *Social Science and Medicine, 61,* 1495–1504.

Kristeva, J. (1980). *Desire in language: A semiotic approach to literature and art.* New York: Columbia University Press.

Kristeva, J. (1984). *Revolution in poetic language.* Columbia: Columbia University Press.

Kristeva, J. (1986a). The system and the speaking subject. In T. Moi (Ed.), *The Kristeva Reader* (pp. 24–33). Oxford: Basil Blackwell.

Kristeva, J. (1986b). Stabat mater. In T. Moi (Ed.), *The Kristeva reader* (pp. 160–186). Oxford: Basil Blackwell.

Kruger, L.-M. and Schoombie, C. (2010). The other side of caring: Abuse in a South African maternity ward. *Journal of Reproductive and Infant Psychology, 28* (1), 84–101.

LaChance Adams, S. and Lundquist, C. (2013). (Eds.). *Coming to life: Philosophies of pregnancy, childbirth and mothering.* New York: Fordham University Press.

Lamaze, F. (1958). *Painless childbirth.* London: Burke.

Lankshear, G., Ettore, E. and Mason, D. (2005). Decision-making, uncertainty and risk: Exploring the complexity of work processes in NHS delivery suites. *Health, Risk and Society, 7* (4), 361–377.

Latour, B. (2005). *Reassembling the social: An introduction to actor-network-theory.* Oxford: Oxford University Press.

Law, J. (2000). On the subject of the object: Narrative, technology, and interpellation. *Configurations, 8* (1), 1–29.

Lazarus, E. (1997). What do women want? Issues of choice, control, and class in American pregnancy and childbirth. In R. Davis-Floyd and C. Sargent (Eds.), *Childbirth and authoritative knowledge* (pp. 132–158). Berkeley: University of California Press.

Leavitt, J. (1986). *Brought to bed: Childbearing in America, 1750–1950.* New York: Oxford University Press.

Leder, D. (1990). *The absent body.* Chicago: Chicago University Press.

Leder, D. (1992). A tale of two bodies: The Cartesian corpse and the lived body. In D. Leder (Ed.), *The body in medical thought and practice* (pp. 117–129). Dordrecht: Kluwer Academic.

Leifer, M. (1977). Psychological changes accompanying pregnancy and motherhood. *Genetic Psychology Monographs, 95,* 55–96.

Lewis, J. (1983). Maternal health in the English aristocracy: Myths and realities, 1790–1840. *Journal of Social History, 17* (1), 97–114.

Lindgren, H., Rådestad, I., Christensson, K., Wally-Bystrom, K. and Hildingsson, I. (2008). Perceptions of risk and risk management among 735 women who opted for a home birth. *Midwifery, 26,* 163–172.

Lintott, S. and Sander-Staudt, M. (2012). (Eds.). *Philosophical inquiries into pregnancy, childbirth, and mothering.* New York: Routledge.

Longhurst, R. (2005). (Ad)dressing pregnant bodies in New Zealand: Clothing, fashion, subjectivities and spatialities. *Gender, Place and Culture, 12* (4), 433–446.

Longhurst, R. (2006). A pornography of birth: Crossing moral boundaries. *ACME: An International Journal E-Journal for Critical Geographies, 5* (2), 209–229.

Longhurst, R. (2009). Youtube: A new space for birth? *Feminist Review, 93,* 46–63.

Lugones, M. (2007). Heterosexualism and the colonial/modern gender system. *Hypatia, 22* (1), 186–219.

Lupton, D. (1997). Foucault and the medicalisation critique. In A. Petersen and R. Bunton (Eds.), *Foucault, health and medicine* (pp. 94–110). London: Routledge.

Lupton, D. (1999a). (Ed). *Risk and sociocultural theory.* Cambridge: Cambridge University Press.

Lupton, D. (1999b). Risk and the ontology of pregnant embodiment. In D. Lupton (Ed.), *Risk and sociocultural theory* (pp. 59–85). Cambridge: Cambridge University Press.

Lupton, D. and Schmied, V. (2013). Splitting bodies/selves: Women's concepts of embodiment at the moment of birth. *Sociology of Health and Illness, 35* (6), 828–841.

Lyerly, A. (2006). Shame, gender, birth. *Hypatia, 21* (1), 101–118.

Lyerly, A. (2012) Ethics and 'normal birth'. *Birth, 39* (4), 315–317.

McAfee, N. (2004). *Julia Kristeva.* New York: Routledge.

Macdonald, M. (2006). Gender expectations: Natural bodies and natural births in the new midwifery in Canada. *Medical Anthropology Quarterly, 20* (2), 235–256.

McKendy, J. (2006). 'I'm very careful about that': Narrative and agency of men in prison. *Discourse and Society, 17* (4), 473–502.

McLaren, M. (2002). *Feminism, Foucault and embodied subjectivity.* New York: State University of New York Press.

Macleod, C. and Howell, S. (2015). Public foetal images and the regulation of middle-class pregnancy in the online media: A view from South Africa. *Culture, Health and Sexuality, 17* (10), 1207–1220.

MacLure, M. (2013). Researching without representation? Language and materiality in post-qualitative methodology. *International Journal of Qualitative Studies in Education, 26* (6), 658–667.

Maher, J. (2003). Rethinking women's birth experience: Medical frameworks and personal narratives. *Hecate, 29* (2), 140–152.

Malacrida, C. and Boulton, T. (2012). Women's perceptions of childbirth 'choices': Competing discourses of motherhood, sexuality, and selflessness. *Gender and Society, 26,* 748–772.

Malacrida, C. and Boulton, T. (2014). The best laid plans? Women's choices, expectations and experiences in childbirth. *Health, 8* (1), 41–59.

Manion, J. (2003). Girls blush, sometimes: Gender, moral agency, and the problem of shame. *Hypatia, 18,* 21–41.

Mardorossian, C. (2003). Laboring women, coaching men: Masculinity and childbirth education in the contemporary United States. *Hypatia, 18* (3), 113–134.

Martin, E. (1987). *The woman in the body: A cultural analysis of reproduction.* Milton Keynes: Open University Press.

Martin, K. (2003). Giving birth like a girl. *Gender and Society, 17* (1), 54–72.

Massey, L. (2005). Pregnancy and pathology: Picturing pregnancy in eighteenth-century obstetric atlases. *Art Bulletin, LXXXVII* (1), 73–91.

Mathai, M. (2011). To ensure maternal mortality is reduced, quality of care needs to be monitored and improved alongside increasing skilled delivery coverage rates. *British Journal of Obstetrics and Gynaeology, 118* (s2), 12–14.

Mies, M. (2014). *Patriarchy and accumulation on a world scale: Women in the international division of labor.* London: Zed Books (original work published 1986).

Michaelson, K. (1988). (Ed). *Childbirth in America: Anthropological perspectives.* Massachusetts: Bergin & Gavey.

Miller, A. (2009). Midwife to myself: Birth narratives among women choosing unassisted homebirth. *Sociological Inquiry, 79* (1), 51–74.

Miller, A. and Shriver, T. (2012). Women's childbirth preferences and practices in the United States. *Social Science and Medicine, 75,* 709–716.

Mohoto, L. (2015). Theatrical strategies of storytelling, bearing witness and testimony for another: An examination of two South African plays. *South African Theatre Journal, 28* (1), 78–87.

Mol, A. (2002). *The body multiple: Ontology in medical practice.* Durham: Duke University Press.

Moodley, J., Pattinson, R., Fawcus, S., Schoon, M., Moran, N. and Shweni, P. (2014). The confidential enquiries into maternal deaths in South Africa: A case study. *British Journal of Obstetrics and Gynaecology, 121* (S4), 53–60.

Moore, R. (2013). Reinventing ethnopoetics. *Journal of Folklore Research, 50* (1–3), 13–39.

Morgan, K. and Thapar-Björkert, S. (2006). 'I'd rather you lay me on the floor and started kicking me': Understanding symbolic violence in everyday life. *Women's Studies International Forum, 29* (5), 441–452.

Moscucci, O. (1990). *The science of woman: Gynaecology and gender in England, 1800–1929.* Cambridge: Cambridge University Press.

Moyzakitis, W. (2004). Exploring women's descriptions of distress and/or trauma in childbirth from a feminist perspective. *Evidence-Based Midwifery, 2* (1), 8–14.

Mozingo, N., Davis, M., Thomas, S. and Droppelman, P. (2002). 'I felt violated': Women's experiences of childbirth-associated anger. *The American Journal of Maternal Child Nursing, 27* (6), 342–348.

Mselle, L., Kohi, T., Mvungi, A., Evjen-Olsen, B. and Moland, K. (2011). Waiting for attention and care: Birthing accounts of women in rural Tanzania who developed obstetric fistula as an outcome of labor. *BMC Pregnancy and Childbirth, 11,* 75.

Müller, M. (2015). Assemblages and actor-networks: Rethinking socio-material power, politics and space. *Geography Compass, 9* (1), 27–41.

Naidoo, N. and Moodley, J. (2009). Rising rates of caesarean sections: An audit of caesarean sections in specialist private practice. *South African Family Practice, 51* (3), 254–258.

Nash, M. (2012). *Making 'postmodern' mothers: Pregnant embodiment, baby bumps and body image.* Basingstoke: Palgrave Macmillan.

Nelson, H. (2001). *Damaged identities, narrative repair.* New York: Cornell University Press.

Nelson, M. (1983). Working-class women, middle-class women, and models of childbirth. *Social Problems, 30* (3), 284–297.

Nicolson, P. (1998). *Postnatal depression: Psychology, science and the transition to motherhood.* London: Routledge.

Nicolson, P. (1999). The myth of the maternal instinct: Feminism, evolution and the case of postnatal depression. *Psychology, Evolution and Gender, 1* (2), 161–181.

Nilsson, C. (2014). The delivery room: Is it a safe place? A hermeneutic analysis of women's negative birth experiences. *Sexual and Reproductive Healthcare, 5* (4), 199–204.

Nilsson, C., Bondas, T. and Lundgren, I. (2010). Previous birth experience in women with intense fear of childbirth. *Journal of Obstetrical, Gynecological and Neonatal Nursing, 39,* 298–309.

Oakley, A. (1980). *Women confined: Towards a sociology of childbirth.* Oxford: Martin Robertsen.

Ochs, E. and Capps, L. (1996). Narrating the self. *Annual Review of Anthropology, 25,* 19–43.

Ochs, E. and Capps, L. (2001). *Living narrative: Creating lives in everyday storytelling.* Cambridge, MA: Harvard University Press.

O'Dell, T. and Willim, R. (2013). Transcription and the senses. *The Senses and Society, 8* (3), 314–334.

Olde, E., Van der Hart, O., Kleber, R., Von Son, M., Wijen, H. and Pop, V. (2005). Peritraumatic dissociation and emotions as predictors of PTSD following childbirth. *Journal of Trauma and Dissociation, 6* (3), 125–142.

Oliver, K. (1993). *Reading Kristeva: Unraveling the double-bind.* Bloomington: Indiana University Press.

Olofsson, A., Zim, J., Griffin, G., Nygren, K., Cebulla, A. and Hannah-Moffat, K. (2014). The mutual constitution of risk and inequalities: Intersectional risk theory. *Health, Risk and Society, 16* (5), 417–430.

Park-Fuller, L. (2000). Performing absence: The staged personal narrative as testimony. *Text and Performance Quarterly, 20* (1), 20–42.

Pérez D'Gregorio, R. (2010). Obstetric violence: A new legal term introduced in Venezuala. *International Journal of Gynecology and Obstetrics, 111,* 201–202.

Pickering, A. (1995). *The mangle of practice: Time, agency, and science.* Chicago: Chicago University Press.

Pickles, C. (2015). Eliminating abusive 'care': A criminal law response to obstetric violence in South Africa. *South African Crime Quarterly, 54,* 5–15.

Pitts-Taylor, V. (2016). *The brain's body: Neuroscience and corporeal politics.* Durham: Duke University Press.

Pollock, D. (1999). *Telling bodies, performing birth: Everyday narratives of childbirth.* New York: Columbia University Press.

Possamai-Inesedy, A. (2006). Confining risk: Choice and responsibility in childbirth in a risk society. *Health Sociology Review, 15,* 406–414.

Pregnancy Mortality Surveillance System, 2016. (2017). Centers for Disease Prevention and Control. Accessed 23 July 2017. www.cdc.gov/reproductivehealth/maternalin fanthealth/pmss.html

Puar, J. (2007). *Terrorist assemblages: Homonationalism in queer times.* Durham: Duke University Press.

Puar, J. (2012). 'I would rather be a cyborg than a goddess': Becoming intersectional in assemblage theory. *philoSOPHIA, 2* (1), 49–66.

Pullen, S. (2015). 'I am one of *those* women': Exploring testimonial performances of stillbirth in/as intervention, support and advocacy. Unpublished Doctoral dissertation: Arizona State University.

Purdy, L. (2001). Medicalization, medical necessity, and feminist medicine. *Bioethics, 15* (3), 248–261.

Pylypa, J. (1998). Power and bodily practice: Applying the work of Foucault to an anthropology of the body. *Arizona Anthropologist, 13,* 21–36.

Rabinow, P. and Rose, N. (2006). Biopower today. *BioSocieties, 1,* 195–217.

Raphael-Leff, J. (1991). *Psychological processes of childbearing.* London: Chapman and Hall.

Raphael-Leff, J. (1993). *Pregnancy: The inside story.* London: Karnac Books.

Rattner, D. (2008). Humanizing childbirth care: Brief theoretical framework. *Interface, 13* (1), 385–392.

Rattner, D., Abreu, I., Araujo, M. and Santos, A. (2007). Humanizing childbirth to reduce maternal and neonatal mortality: A national effort in Brazil. In R. Davis-Floyd, L. Barclay, B.-A Daviss and J. Tritten (Eds.), *Birth models that work* (pp. 385–413). Berkeley: University of California Press.

Reiger, K. and Dempsey, R. (2006). Performing birth in a culture of fear: an embodied crisis of late modernity. *Health Sociology Review, 15* (4), 364–373.

Rich, A. (1986). *Of woman born: Motherhood as experience and institution.* New York: W.W. Norton and Company.

Root, R. and Browner, C. (2001). Practices of the pregnant self: Compliance with, and resistance to, prenatal norms. *Culture, Medicine and Psychiatry, 25* (2), 195–223.

Rose, N. (2001) The politics of life itself. *Theory, Culture and Society, 18* (6), 1–30.

Rossiter, K. (2017). Pushing ecstasy: Neoliberalism, childbirth, and the making of mama economicus. *Women's Studies, 46* (1), 41–59.

Rothberg, A. and Macleod, H. (2005). Private sector caesarean sections in perspective. *South African Medical Journal, 95* (4), 54–61.

Rothman, B.K. (1982). *In labor: Women and power in the birthplace.* New York: W.W. Norton and Company.

Sadler, M., Santos, M., Ruiz-Berdún, D., Leiva Rojas, G., Skoko, E., Gillen, P. and Clausen, J. (2016). Moving beyond disrespect and abuse: Addressing the structural dimensions of obstetric violence. *Reproductive Health Matters, 24,* 47–55.

Saisto, T. and Halmesmäki, E. (2003). Fear of childbirth: A neglected dilemma. *Acta Obstetricia Gyaecologica Scandinavica, 82* (3), 201–208.

Sawicki, J. (1991). *Disciplining Foucault: Feminism, body and the body.* New York: Routledge.

Saxbe, D. (2017). Birth of a new perspective? A call for biopsychosocial research on childbirth. *Current Directions in Psychological Science, 26* (1), 81–86.

Sbisà, M. (1996). The feminine subject and female body in discourse about childbirth. *The European Journal of Women's Studies, 3*, 363–376.

Scamell, M. (2011). The swan effect in midwifery talk and practice: A tension between normality and the language of risk. *Sociology of Health and Illness, 33* (7), 987–1001.

Scamell, M. and Alaszewski, A. (2012). Fateful moments and the categorisation of risk: Midwifery practice and the ever-narrowing window of normality during childbirth. *Health, Risk and Society, 14* (2), 207–221.

Schiebinger, L. (2013). *Nature's body: Gender in the making of modern science.* New Brunswick: Rutgers University Press (original work published 1993).

Schmied, V. and Lupton, D. (2001a). The externality of the inside: Body images of pregnancy. *Nursing Inquiry, 8* (1), 32–40.

Schmied, V. and Lupton, D. (2001b). Blurring the boundaries: Breastfeeding and maternal subjectivity. *Sociology of Health and Illness, 23* (2), 234–250.

Schneider, H., le Marcic, F., Grard, J., Penn-Kekana, L., Blaaw, D. and Fassin, D. (2010). Negotiating care: Patient tactics at an urban South African hospital. *Journal of Health Services Research and Policy, 15* (3), 137–142.

Schroll, A.-M., Kjaergaard, H. and Midtgaard, J. (2013). Encountering abuse in health care: Lifetime experiences in postnatal women—a qualitative study. *BMC Pregnancy and Childbirth, 13*, 74.

Searle, C. (1965). *The history of the development of nursing in South Africa 1652–1960: A sociohistorical survey.* Pretoria: The South African nursing association.

Sedgwick, E. (1993). *Tendencies.* Durham: Duke University Press.

Segal, L. (1994). *Straight sex: Rethinking the politics of pleasure.* Berkeley: University of California Press.

Seibold, C., Licqurish, S., Rolls, C. and Hopkins, F. (2010). 'Lending the space': Midwives perceptions of birth space and clinical risk management. *Midwifery, 26*, 526–531.

Shabot, S. (2016). Making loud bodies 'feminine': A feminist-phenomenological analysis of obstetric violence. *Human Studies, 39* (2), 231–247.

Sharpe, S. (1999). Bodily speaking: Spaces and experiences of childbirth. In E. Teather (Ed.), *Embodied geographies: Spaces, bodies and rites of passage* (pp. 91–103). London: Routledge.

Shaw, R. (2002). The ethics of the birth plan in childbirth management practices. *Feminist Theory, 3* (2), 131–149.

Shaw, R. and Kitzinger, C. (2007). Problem presentation and advice-giving on a home-birth helpline: A feminist conversation analytic study. *Feminism and Psychology, 17* (2), 203– 213.

Shereshefsky, P. and Yarrow, L. (1973). (Eds.) *Psychological aspects of a first pregnancy and early postnatal adaptation.* New York: Raven Press.

Shilling, C. (1993). *The body and social theory.* London: Sage.

Shorter, E. (1982). *A history of women's bodies.* New York: Basic Books.

Simonds, W. (2002). Watching the clock: Keeping time during pregnancy, birth, and postpartum experiences. *Social Science and Medicine, 55*, 559–570.

Skeggs, B. (1997). *Formations of class and gender: Becoming respectable.* London: Sage.

Smith-Oka, V. (2015). Microaggressions and the reproduction of social inequalities in medical encounters in Mexico. *Social Science and Medicine, 143*, 9–16.

Soet, J., Brack, G. and Dilorio, C. (2003). Prevalence and predictors of women's experience of psychological trauma during childbirth. *Birth, 30* (1), 36–46.

South African Demographic and Health Survey, 2003. (2007). Department of Health, Medical Research Council. Pretoria: Department of Health.

South African Demograhic and Health Survey, 2016. (2017). Department of Health, Medical Research Council. Pretoria: Department of Health. Accessed 23 July 2017. www.statssa.gov.za/publications/Report%2003-00-09/Report%2003-00-092016.pdf

Spangler, S. (2011). 'To open oneself is a poor woman's trouble': Embodied inequality and childbirth in south-central Tanzania. *Medical Anthropology Quarterly, 25* (4), 479–498.

Statistics SA. (2013). *Gender statistics in South Africa,* 2011. Pretoria, South Africa. Accessed 23 July 2017. www.statssa.gov.za/publications/Report-03-10-05/Report-03-10-052011.pdf

Statistics SA. (2014). Poverty trends in South Africa: An examination of absolute poverty between 2006 and 2011. Pretoria, South Africa. Accessed 23 July 2017. https://beta2.statssa.gov.za/publications/Report-03-10-06/Report-03-10-06March2014.pdf

Stearns, C. (1999). Breastfeeding and the good maternal body. *Gender and Society, 13* (3), 308–325.

Stephens, J. (2004). Beyond binaries in motherhood research. *Family Matters, 69,* 88–93.

Stern, D. and Bruschweiler-Stern, N. (1998). *The birth of a mother.* New York: Basic Books.

Swahnberg, K., Thapar-Björkert, B. and Berterö, C. (2007). Nullified: Women's perceptions of being abused in health care. *Journal of Psychosomatic Obstetrics and Gynecology, 28* (3), 161–167.

Tanassi, L. (2004). Compliance as strategy: The importance of personalized relations in obstetric practice. *Social Science and Medicine, 59,* 2053–2069.

Taylor, J. (2000). Of sonograms and baby prams: Prenatal diagnosis, pregnancy, and consumption. *Feminist Studies, 26* (2), 391–418.

Taylor, J. (2008). *The public life of the fetal sonogram: Technology, consumption, and the politics of reproduction.* New Jersey: Rutgers University Press.

Taylor, J., Layne, L. and Wozniak, D. (2004). (Eds.). *Consuming motherhood.* New Jersey: Rutgers University Press.

The Lancet Series (2016). Maternal health: An executive summary for *The Lancet's* series. Accessed 23 July 2017. www.thelancet.com/pb/assets/raw/Lancet/stories/series/maternal-health-2016/mathealth2016-exec-summ.pdf

Thomas, L. (2003). *Politics of the womb: Women, reproduction and the state in Kenya.* Berkeley: University of California Press.

Thompson, C. (2003). Natural health discourse and the therapeutic production of consumer resistance. *Sociological Quarterly, 44* (1), 81–107.

Thomson, G. and Downe, S. (2008). Widening the trauma discourse: The link between childbirth and experiences of abuse. *Journal of Psychosomatic Obstetrics and Gynaecology, 29* (4), 268–273.

Tritten, J. (2009). Birth is a human rights issue. *Midwifery Today, 92.*

Tshibangu, K., de Jongh, M., de Villiers, D., du Toit, J. and Shah, S. (2002). Incidence and outcome of caesarean sections in the private sector: A 3-year experience at Pretoria Gynaecological Hospital. *South African Medical Journal, 92* (12), 956–959.

Tyler, I. (2011). Pregnant beauty: Maternal femininities under neoliberalism. In R. Gill and C. Scharff (Eds.), *New femininities: Postfeminism, neoliberalism and subjectivity* (pp. 21– 36). Basingstoke: Palgrave Macmillan.

Turner, B. (1984). *The body and society: Explorations in social theory.* London: Sage.

Ussher, J. (1989). *The psychology of the female body.* London: Routledge.

Ussher, J. (2006). *Managing the monstrous feminine: Regulating the reproductive body.* London: Routledge.

Van den Broek, N. and Graham, W. (2009). Quality of care for maternal and newborn health: The neglected agenda. *British Journal of Obstetrics and Gynaecology, 116* (s1), 18–21.

Van der Tuin, I. (2014). Diffraction as a methodology for feminist onto-epistemology: On encountering Chantal Chawaf and posthuman interpellation. *Parallax, 20* (3), 231–244.

VandeVusse, L. (1999). Decision-making in analyses of women's birth stories. *Birth, 26* (1), 43–50.

Viisainen, K. (2000). The moral dangers of home birth: Parents' perceptions of risk in home birth in Finland. *Sociology of Health and Illness, 22* (6), 792–814.

Vissing, H. (2017). A perfect birth: The birth rights movement and the idealization of birth. In E. Toronto, J. Ponder, K. Davisson and M. Kelber Kelly (Eds.), *A womb of her own: Women's struggles for sexual and reproductive autonomy* (pp. 171–183). London: Routledge.

Vogel, J., Bohren, M., Tuncalp, Ö., Oladapo, O. and Gülmezoglu, A. (2016). Promoting respect and preventing mistreatment during childbirth. *British Journal of Obstetrics and Gynaecology, 123* (5), 671–674.

Wagner, M. (2001). Fish can't see water: The need to humanize birth. *International Journal of Gynecology and Obstetrics,* 75, s25–37.

Waldenström, U. (1999). Experience of labor and birth in 1111 women. *Journal of Psychosomatic Research, 47* (5), 471–482.

Waldenström, U., Hildingsson, I., Rubertsson, C. and Rådestad, I. (2004). A negative birth experience: Prevalence and risk factors in a national sample. *Birth, 31* (1), 17–27.

Walsh, D. (2010). Childbirth embodiment: Problematic aspects of current understandings. *Social Science and Medicine, 32* (3), 486–501.

Warren, S. and Brewis, J. (2004). Mind over matter? Examining the experience of pregnancy. *Sociology, 38* (2), 219–236.

Weaver, J. (1998). Choice, control and decision-making in labor. In S. Clements and L. Page (Eds.), *Psychological perspectives on pregnancy and childbirth* (pp. 81–99). Edinburgh: Churchill Livingstone.

Williams, S. and Bendelow, G. (1998). *The lived body: Sociological themes, embodied issues.* London: Routledge.

Wolf, A. (2013). Metaphysical violence and medicalized childbirth. *International Journal of Applied Philosophy, 27* (1), 101–111.

World Health Organization. (2014). The prevention and elimination of disrespect and abuse during facility-based childbirth. Accessed 24 July 2017. http://apps.who.int/iris/bitstream/10665/134588/1/WHO_RHR_14.23_eng.pdf?ua=1&ua=1

Wynn, F. (2002). The early relationship of mother and pre-infant: Merleau-Ponty and pregnancy. *Nursing Philosophy,* 3, 4–14.

Young, I.-M. (1990a). *Throwing like a girl and other essays in feminist philosophy and social theory.* Bloomington: Indiana University Press.

Young, I.-M. (1990b). *Justice and the politics of difference.* Princeton: Princeton University Press.

Zadoroznyj, M. (1999). Social class, social selves and social control in childbirth. *Sociology of Health & Illness, 21* (3), 267–289.

Zadoroznyj, M. (2001). Birth and the 'reflexive consumer': Trust, risk, and medical dominance in obstetric encounters. *Journal of Sociology, 37* (2), 117–139.

Žižek, S. (2008). *Violence: Six sideways reflections.* New York: Picador.

Zukin, S. and Maguire, J. (2004). Consumers and consumption. *Annual Review of Sociology,* 30, 173–197

Appendix 1
RESEARCH NOTE

In this note, I provide a brief outline of the research projects on which this book is based and contextualize the research process. The voices that vitalize this book are drawn from 85 interviews conducted with 64 South African women. These interviews were gathered over many years and as part of two research projects. In the first study, 29 women participated. This research project (my PhD) explored 'agency' in relation to birth and focused predominantly on the experiences of women planning to give birth at home or via an elective caesarean section. In this study, 24 of the women took part in pre- and post-birth interviews. Two women were interviewed once post-birth and three women participated in email correspondence. Most of the 29 women who participated in the first study were white and middle class (n = 27). A total of 15 women had a planned homebirth, 12 chose to birth via elective caesarean section, one woman had an emergency caesarean section and one gave birth vaginally in a private hospital. In the second research project, 35 women who had given birth in the public sector were interviewed shortly after giving birth (three days to four weeks postpartum). All of these participants were black, low-income and living in various informal settlements across the Western Cape region of South Africa. Of these women, 27 gave birth vaginally, while 8 had emergency caesarean sections, 16 women gave birth in MOU settings and 17 in public hospitals. One woman gave birth at home with no skilled caregiver and another gave birth while in transit to health facilities. In both research projects, most interviews were conducted in women's homes, which included shacks, backyard dwellings, council flats and houses. Women's homes ranged from mansions in some of the richest suburbs in Cape Town to shacks with no electricity or basic furniture and with sand as floors. One woman was homeless and interviewed in a woman's shelter. Women were recruited with help from private midwives, letters to local community newspapers, visits to private hospital antenatal classes and with the assistance of a local non-governmental organization (NGO) that ran a community home-based visiting program for vulnerable mothers in informal settlements. The 64 women whose stories are represented in this book were thus racially and socioeconomically diverse; 27 women were white and 37 women were black. Of these, 30 women were of mixed racial descent (locally known as 'coloured') while 7 were black African. All of the women who participated provided informed consent and are referred to in the book via pseudonyms. I conducted, transcribed and analyzed all of the interviews.

The research journeys undertaken in these two projects were very different. In the first study, I interviewed predominantly affluent, highly educated (often professional) and predominantly white women. I visited warm, comfortable and cosy homes, was treated as a friend and given tea and snacks. Interviews were largely conversational and women spoke at length and with clear enjoyment about their experiences of pregnancy, birth and early mothering. Although I was an outsider in some respects (i.e. I have never been pregnant, given birth or mothered a child), sociomaterial similarities (race, class, gender and education) with most of these participants meant that the interviewing process was relatively smooth and generally enjoyable. I also conducted two interviews with most of these participants (pre- and post-birth) and thus was able to form meaningful relationships with many of the women that I interviewed.

The second research project was very different. Given the difficulties of finding participants who inhabited very different social worlds to myself (i.e. poor women attending public sector services), I collaborated with a local NGO to recruit suitable women. This meant working with community workers based in various informal settlements across the Western Cape who very kindly informed potential participants about the project and set up interviews. The logistics of these interviews were often very difficult as participants lived in high density and poverty-stricken areas (i.e. 'townships') characterized by high levels of violence. As a young, white woman unfamiliar with this terrain, it was not safe for me to negotiate these spaces alone. As a result, community workers accompanied me to women's homes, helping me to traverse unfamiliar zones in which gang warfare was a daily reality. The 35 women interviewed in this project lived in 10 different informal settlements in the wider Cape Town metropole, including: Manenberg, Heideveld, Hanover Park, Imizamo Yethu, Hangberg, Lavender Hill, Nyanga, New Crossroads, Gugulethu and Mitchell's Plain. Interviews with these women were punctuated with difficulties, discomforts, disruptions and dangers. I felt my difference viscerally as I navigated these neighborhoods and interviewing spaces. Language was often a problem given that I do not speak isiXhosa (the dominant local African language). As a result, interviews with first-language isiXhosa speakers (n = 7) were conducted in English (if women consented to this). The majority of women (n = 28) were, however, first-language Afrikaans speakers. As I am relatively proficient in this language, I was able to conduct these interviews in Afrikaans and translate the interview transcripts into English. Given the multiple differences between myself and participants (language, race, class position, education), these interviews were often riddled with misunderstandings and strains. However, there were also moments of connection, warmth and laughter and some participants seemed to enjoy being interviewed. Given that my spoken Afrikaans is relatively poor, many women were also amused at my attempts to speak their language. This often lightened the mood and sometimes worked to usefully disrupt my positionality as educated and 'expert' interviewer.

Appendix 2

TRANSCRIPTION NOTATION

*	Undecipherable words
(*)	Short pause (less than 2 seconds)
(**)	Long pause (2–3 seconds)
(***)	Very long pause (more than 4 seconds)
(. . .)	Words omitted
You(r)	Completion of word in bracket
Massive (in bold)	Words spoken loudly
. . .	Speech trails off
#	One person talks over the other
Good thing (italicized)	Words spoken slowly
<u>No</u> (underlined)	Words that are emphasized
^^Oh yes^^	Words spoken with laughter in the voice
<u>Tiny</u> (bolded, underlined and italicized)	Words spoken loudly, slowly and with emphasis
↑Oh my word↑	High-pitched words
{I don't know}	Whispered
<u>Definitely</u> (bolded and underlined)	Words spoken loudly and with emphasis
[doctor]	Explanatory material
OH NO (capitalized)	Words shouted out
X	Details omitted to protect anonymity

INDEX

abjection 46, 75; and birthing body 82–88, 100, 123, 202

acts of telling 18–19, 131, 142–150

affect 11, 14–15, 21, 83–85, 99, 111, 126, 128, 130, 132, 168, 171, 192–196, 199

affective politics 193–196, 199

agency 9, 11–12, 39–42, 51–53, 58–59, 66, 68–70, 73, 97, 100, 105, 107–109, 113–117, 130, 138–141, 143, 147–149, 169, 196–201

agential realism 14

Althusser, Louis 20–21

assemblage 11–13, 123, 130, 131, 132, 139, 171, 193–194, 196–197

Barad, Karen 11, 12, 14–15

biomedical birth see birth

biomedical body 25–27

biomedical power see power

biopower 77, 97

birth: and access to information 64–68, 71; Africa 7, 28–19; as biological event 25–26; biomedical birth 9–10, 25, 132; colonial myths 28–30; and consumerism 40–41; and culture 25–26; and femininity 44–46; and human rights 37–38; idealizations 4, 34–36, 170, 192; injustice 4, 163–164, 169, 201; mistreatment 6, 75, 82, 93, 101, 109, 113, 128–129, 161–168; natural birth 28–30, 64, 69, 71, 76, 110, 200, 201; 'normal' birth 4, 34–35, 52, 69, 170, 195, 201; and psychoanalysis 32–33; and psychology 30–33; and race 28–30,

36, 63, 74; and sexuality 85–86, 118, 122–123; trauma 4, 32, 65, 89, 102, 112, 114, 118, 143

birth assemblage 51–53, 58, 60, 62, 71, 73–74, 107–109, 111–112, 121, 123, 128, 130, 135, 139, 140, 169, 171, 196–199, 200, 202

birth rights movement 35

birth satisfaction 32

birth stories 13, 15, 19, 50, 72, 131, 133–139, 143, 144, 200–201

birth violence see obstetric violence; see also distress

birthing body: biomedical 25–27, 50; biomedical power 43–44; 'body-in-labor' 47, 60, 70, 113, 115, 145; body self relations 47–49, 69–70; embodied agency 48, 52, 69, 70, 71–72, 97, 113–117, 130, 138–140, 148, 149, 169, 196–198;femininity 44–46; loud 33, 46, 113, 115–116, 148, 196, 198, 202; natural 26, 30, 36, 69, 81, 98; as object 56, 66, 87, 105–107, 117, 129–130, 149; physiological 35; psychofleshy aspects 33, 46–49, 66, 82, 113, 115, 126, 142, 149, 168–169, 196, 199, 202; and race 28–30, 123; and risk 75, 82, 100; studies 47–49; technocratic 75; vulnerable 82–88, 118; why? 1–3

bodies: Foucauldian approach 8–10; and language 16–18; new materialism 10–13; reproductive 46–47; and storytelling 19–20

caesarean section 5–6, 75–78, 81–82, 84–85, 111, 126–127, 150–160, 193–194, 201
care 87–90, 97, 99, 128, 139, 199
choice 2, 9, 39–42, 49, 61, 91–92, 106–107, 109–113, 201, 202
coloniality of power 28, 29, 90
control 87, 88, 100, 148
counternarrative 134, 143

Dick-Read, Grantly 29–30
diffraction 3, 14–15, 16
diffractive methodology 15
dignity 75, 81–85, 87–88, 90, 95, 100, 117–121, 122, 125, 130, 198–199
discourse: discursive practice 17; and relation to materiality 16–17
distress 150–161, 169, 194–195
docile bodies 8, 10, 42–44, 107–109, 130
double consciousness 86, 88
dualism 1–2, 25, 27, 192; and biomedical bodies 25–27; and non-dualism 11

embodied ethics 199, 203
embodied inequality 4–7, 29, 41, 90, 96, 107, 120, 197
embodied oppression 113, 123, 127, 130, 148, 197, 202
embodied subject 15–17
embodied telling 142–150
embodied politics 192, 203
enactment 12, 13, 196, 197
entanglement 12, 14, 15, 111, 126, 139, 143, 150, 197
ethnopoetics 18
expectations 53, 60, 68–69

fear of childbirth 32
femininity 44–46, 86
feminism and birth 25–27
Foucault, Michel 3, 8–10, 42–44, 50, 91, 95–97, 108
Frank, Arthur 3, 19–21, 131, 143, 150, 151, 158, 162
free birth 30, 36, 64
Friedman's curve 52

gentle violence 104, 108, 112, 127, 129–130, 201
geopolitics of birth 3–4, 6–7, 26–27, 29, 33–34, 38–42, 74, 90, 102, 170
Gilligan, Carol 21, 131, 151
good birth 193–195, 198, 203
good patient 107–109, 116

Haraway, Donna 12, 15, 16, 18, 20, 143
homebirth 30, 52–54, 57, 59, 60, 64, 68–70, 71–73, 75, 78–82, 84, 87, 88–90, 100, 133–137, 139–140, 144–145, 149, 196, 198
humanizing birth 38–39
humor 133–139, 147, 168

ideologies 20, 84, 201
ideology critique 20
'I poems' 21, 144, 151–157, 158–160
interference patterns 12, 15, 16, 18, 20
interpellation 20–21
intersectionality 7, 12–13, 39, 41, 51, 103, 203
invisibility 74, 81, 91, 95–99, 101, 194, 197, 200
intra-action 12, 14, 96, 111, 117, 130, 140, 200, 201–202

Kristeva, Julia 3, 16–18, 83, 143

language: and bodies 16–17, 142–143; decentering 17; as material force 16; and new materialism 17–18;
Leder, Drew 113
listening guide 21, 151
Lugones, Maria 28

mangle 12, 193
master narratives 70, 132–133, 136, 143
maternal mortality rate: global 4; South Africa 4–6, 90
maternity 31, 77, 111
maternity care 170–171, 195, 203
medicalization 25–27, 49, 71–72, 73, 160; and race 28–30, 61–64
methodology 18–21, 131–133, 142–143
Mol, Annemarie 2, 24, 202

narrative: and bodies 20, 142–150; dialogical narrative analysis 3, 19–21, 131–133; distress 150, 169; and resistance 131–133, 142, 146, 162, 164, 168–169; testimonial 161–168
narrative poems 19, 131, 151–157–160, 171–192
natural birth 28–30, 64, 69, 71, 76, 110, 200, 201
neoliberalism 3, 9, 36, 40–41, 61, 91, 109–110, 112
new materialism 10–15, 143
normal birth 4, 34–35, 52, 69, 170, 195, 201

objectification 88, 100, 105, 114, 115, 117, 149
obstetric violence 7, 27, 38, 102–104
onto-epistemology 13–14
ontological politics 2, 13, 24–25, 39, 193, 202

pain 28–29, 36, 47, 62, 67, 70, 123, 129, 139, 148, 149
panopticon 43, 95, 96, 101
passivity 105–107, 130
patriarchal optics 45, 84, 85–88, 100, 121–123
physiological birth 36
politics of birth: embodied 192–193; feminist: 2, 6–7, 26–27, 39–42; global: 2–3, 33–34, 170; moral 77–82, 120–123; South Africa 201
positive birth 114, 133–140, 143–150, 193–194
post-traumatic stress disorder 32
power 8–10, 195, 200; biomedical power 9, 43–44, 50–51, 71–72, 74, 200; and disciplinary power 8–9, 64, 108; and gender 44–46; and narratives 50–51; biopower 77
posthuman 14
poststructuralism 14
poverty 92–95, 101, 119–120, 124, 146
privacy 75, 82, 85, 87, 100, 118–119, 130
private sector birth 5–6, 57, 64–65, 72, 75, 87–88, 90–91, 95, 100–101, 109–113, 126–127, 130, 135, 149, 158–160, 200–201
psychology and birth 30–33
Puar, Jasbir 12–13
public sector birth 5–6, 53, 55–56, 61–68, 71–72, 74–75, 82, 87–99, 100–101, 105–109, 114–115, 118–129, 133, 137, 141–142, 145, 149–150, 160–168, 200–201

race 5–7, 28–30, 36, 44, 51, 53, 57, 63, 66, 71, 74, 87, 90, 96, 116, 121–123, 130, 197, 199, 202
racialized patriarchy 90, 103, 120, 123, 130, 200
Raphael-Leff, Joan 33
relational assemblage 139–143, 194, 198

relational violence 113, 116, 128
research assemblage 13, 58, 106, 132
resistance 131, 133, 141, 147, 150, 162, 164, 166, 168–169, 202
risk: biomedical 3–4; and bodies 75
risk economies 74, 75 77, 78, 80, 87, 88, 90–92, 96, 100–101, 160
risk politics 74, 90–92, 99, 100, 101
'risks to life' 74, 77, 78, 81, 92, 93, 95, 100, 101
'risks to self' 74–75, 82, 83, 89, 92, 93, 95, 100, 101
risky body 75, 82, 100

safe birth 77, 89, 112
safety 85, 89, 196, 197, 198–199
semiotic 16, 19
shame 81, 82, 84, 87, 92, 95, 100, 120, 121–123, 198
social constructionism 7–8, 13–14; 31; and bodies 8; and discourse determinism 10
social Darwinism 29
South Africa: caesarean section rates 5; demographics 4–5; economic inequality 4–5; health system 4–6; maternal mortality rate 5–6
speaking body 16, 17, 169
sterilization 119–120
structural violence 103, 126, 129
surveillance 43–44, 63, 73, 74, 88, 91, 95–96, 97, 98–99, 148
symbolic 16
symbolic violence 104, 108, 130

technologies of gender 44–46, 86–87
testimonial narratives 161–168
tokophobia 32
transcription 18, 132
transition to motherhood 31
transnational birth activism 42
traumatic birth 4, 32, 65, 89, 102, 112, 114, 118, 143

visibility 43, 45, 64, 74, 85–88, 91, 95–99, 100–101, 197, 202
vulnerability 82–88, 100, 118

Young, Iris Marion 46, 78, 86, 106

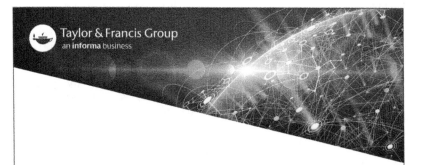